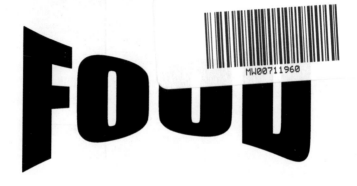

FOOD

is NOT the Boss of Me!

THE JOURNAL

By Elizabeth Bailey Copeland

A day by day guide strengthening you to make healthy eating choices

Published by God's People Ministry, Inc.
(www.godspeopleministry.org)

Printed by Copyworks www.copyworksatlanta.com

Unless otherwise noted, "Scripture quotations taken from the Amplified® Bible, Copyright © 1954, 1958, 1962, 1964, 1965, 1987 by The Lockman Foundation. Used by permission." (www.Lockman.org)

Other scripture references as noted are from the following sources: King James Version (KJV); The New King James Version. Copyright © 1979, 1980, 1982 by Thomas Nelson, Inc. Used by permission. All rights reserved. THE MESSAGE. Copyright © by Eugene H. Peterson, 1993, 1994, 1995, 1996. Used by permission of NavPress Publishing Group.

Copeland, Elizabeth Bailey, 1958—

Library of Congress, Food is NOT the Boss of Me! The Journal Elizabeth Bailey Copeland, Religion, Health
ISBN   978-0-9720304-2-7 (paperback)
1. Devotional – Health 2. Devotional-Calendar

Dedication

It is with great honor that I dedicate this book to my beloved father, the late Willie Frank Bailey.

When my dad was diagnosed with Prostate cancer in his early sixties, I watched as he took ownership of his health. Daddy was a well known, respected and successful businessman in our community. He was a workaholic; an excellent provider for his family; a devout reader; a student of the Word of God; settled in his ways; and a sort of connoisseur of good food!

I recall in our earlier years of growing up, without fail, every winter my dad would purchase a whole cow and a pig to stock my mother's freezer. Yes, food was a huge object in our lives! Every Bailey gathering was assured to have a lavish and delicious meal that my mom, Evelyn Jean Mahaffey Bailey (Ms. Evelyn) had prepared. Even so, on many occasions, as a family, we would frequent restaurants of fine dining.

After his diagnoses, my father drastically changed his mind on how he viewed food and its purpose. His game plan was spelled out in three steps: *1) educating, 2) exercising and 3) eating to live!* He became a responsible steward of his body (temple) and completely changed what and how he ate; amazing everyone and adding years to his life.

My admiration for Daddy grew stronger as I witnessed the discipline, determination and extreme weight loss. Simultaneously, his faith in God and the truth of His Word grew stronger. Of equal importance, he felt better and looked years younger. His doctors were continually amazed.

On February 12, 2001, my Heavenly Father called my earthly father home; to give his body eternal rest. I am thankful for the legacy that my father has left for me. Daddy believed in me and enjoyed reading my writing. He is greatly missed and lovingly remembered.

"I will persist until I succeed."
Willie Frank Bailey
(January 27, 1932- February 12, 2001)

Acknowledgements

Without the continual loving support and encouragement of my husband of 30 years, Jerome Copeland, Sr., this writing would not have been possible. Honey, I appreciate your believing in me. Mostly, I thank you for loving me—unconditionally and being my best friend! In your words, *we are a team!* And I add—*for life!*

My sincere appreciation is extended to my children, Jessica and Jerome, Jr. I am forever grateful for your giving me the true pleasures of being a Mom and keeping me young! I value your candid feedback and suggestions. Thanks for the tireless reading of my work and your openness to dream with me! I await God's awesome plan for your lives to unfold!

To Felecia and David, Tamika and Cornelius, I am privileged to call you my children and honored to be Mom#2!

To my mother, Evelyn Bailey, I thank you for choosing life and loving me. To my mother in love, Nina Copeland, thank you for choosing life for my best friend.

To Bernice Bailey, Omega Bailey and Frankie Wynder, faithful original team members of God's People Ministry (GPM), you believed from the start and continue to do so!

To Pamela Booker, I am forever grateful for your consistent belief in GPM expressed through your support.

To my spiritual father, Pastor Erven A. Kimble; thank you for seeing the vision long before I even knew how to dream.

To Bishop Fritz and Lady Lisa, thank you for the opportunity to prove that it is so!

To those who sustain me in prayer and those who will read this writing, may God bless your labor of love to His saint!

To Mama Kay Simmons (my spiritual mother) and Theresia Ellison Woods, my faithful Monday prayer team—your love continually sustains me. *A threefold cord…keep it moving!*

Foreword

"Food is Not the Boss of Me" is a fresh and powerful concept that far surpasses the typical mindset on diet and exercise. Beth has communicated beautifully that we have an unhealthy attraction to food. She brings a Spiritual solution to this issue that you have never heard before. She has effectively drawn in varying cultures, religious beliefs, and economic backgrounds and how they impact what we think and do. Your life will be forever changed by the Spiritual and practical insight Beth offers!

I have known Beth Copeland for many years and have had the privilege of seeing God do great things through her. She is a very disciplined and faithful woman of God. Her daily walk with God is priority number one. She is a busy woman; yet, she remains committed to her husband, their children and work in the local church. One of the things I admire most about Beth is that she WALKS what she TALKS. She leads by example. Her outstanding example further validates her spoken and written communications. She is a woman of highest integrity with a genuine love for all people. She is a mighty woman of God, a fireball for the Army of God. Beth is an anointed writer and speaker; and, her seminars always take people to higher levels of understanding and revelation.

Beth uses the acronym "RULE" to lay a foundation you will never forget. The way we look at things has everything to do with the person we become. When we view something incorrectly, it becomes a bad seed that produces a bad harvest.

Absorb this book. Meditate on these principles. Take advantage of the accompanying Journal that offers daily structure for keeping yourself on track. Allow yourself to become FREE from the bondage of food addiction once and for all by doing it the right way, God's way! Start putting these tools in place NOW and don't let food ever be the boss of you again!

—First Lady Lisa Musser
Tabernacle International Church, Lawrenceville, GA

Introduction

As the result of a successful 40 day liquid fast, seeking God on a higher level and asking Him for answers to so many challenging and puzzling questions in my life, I was inspired to write the book *Food is NOT the boss of me!* This journal has been created as an accompaniment to the book in an effort to facilitate your success, as you aspire to be the best you!

The background information forthcoming is being included within this journal for the benefit of those that have not had the opportunity to read the introduction to the book:

The day following the close of my fast, I was flabbergasted when the Holy Spirit revealed that I had been delivered from a *'food addiction'*. That comment registered in my spirit; literally, stopping me right in my tracks. I questioned how could it be—*an addiction? Food?* My weight challenges were not included on my list of concerns for my fast; yet, I knew instantly that God was speaking directly to me.

The truth of the matter was that food had subtly controlled me for the length of my life—as far back as I can remember! You see, food was my drug of choice; food was how I got my fix! It seemed as if it was harmless and permissible because it was food and food is needed in order to survive, correct? Yet, it had become my god; because I was unable to control it—*food controlled me!*

My flesh drove my desire for food: telling me what to eat, when to eat it and how much! Even when I would recognize that I was overeating and wanted to stop, my flesh went to war and most often won! I ate to satisfy my flesh, not my need. My eating or not eating, for the most part, was driven by recreation and situation.

However, during the fast, when I subjected myself wholeheartedly to God, resisting the desires of my flesh, through His power, I begin to _rule_ over my flesh; to dominate and take back the reins of my life! *"So be subject to God. Resist the devil [stand firm against him], and he will flee from you."*[1]

Through my submission to God, I received a revelation: I possess the power to rule over my life in every aspect! I begin to understand that I could resist the temptation of unhealthy and unwise food choices and *so much more!* Through caring for my temple, I could be my best for God, bringing Him greater glory and demonstrating my love for Him on a higher level. And, my love for others grew stronger! When I was at my best, it brought me a significant level of empowerment! —I saw things from a new and different perspective; hearing God's voice was clearer and unobstructed. My creativity was pumping; I was productive and I felt victorious!

---

[1] James 4:7

As mentioned in the book and restated here, the freedom that I am experiencing is incredible. I am realizing God and His Word from an elevated perspective. I began to understand that my addiction was comparable to any other—it was unhealthy, crippling and detrimental to my experiencing the quality life that God had designed for me!

Through meditation, I recognized that my deliverance was a divine intervention that is available to others. I am thankful to God for His undying, unconditional love and humbled that He has chosen me to share this dynamic, empowering and life changing journal with you. He has no respect of person, what He has done and is doing for me—He welcomes the opportunity to do the same and even more for you!

This journal has been designed to assist you as you take RULE over your life! The value that you will realize from faithfully maintaining this journal is greater than the best diet, workout routine, 12 step program, and support group or therapy session. You will begin to recognize that you are infused with the power to overcome and be victorious in your journey to becoming the best you!

My dear friend, you were created and destined for greatness! You have been impregnated with supernatural power; to accomplish and do awesome and wonderful things. There is so very much more available that you have not even dreamed of or tapped into! Yet, you must release the baggage that is weighing you down to unleash the optimal you!

Retracing my steps during the fast, I discovered that I had created a simple daily strategy that contributed to my success. My greatest desire is to share with you this unique game plan. You will be challenged to spend time in prayer communicating with God! While being held accountable to be a faithful steward over the most valuable treasures that He has entrusted to you!

Effectively working this journal, in accordance with the outline to follow, provides you an effective tool that is essential for your success in every aspect of your life!

Appropriating the Journal

1)   The day started with a _prayer focus_. This provided the necessary strength to face each day with a 'can do' attitude! My dependency grew more so in this area, than in any other. Aside from my specific initial prayer request at the onset of the fast, most of my time in prayer was intercessory. My focus was directed to particular concerns for the needs of others and/or situations or circumstances locally, nationally or globally. Embracing prayer heighten my prayer life! I developed greater confidence that I was communicating effectively with God. My assurance was His peace and/or response to me. This was my new lifestyle—whether silent or audibly; dedicated or spontaneous; alone or in unison; kneeling or standing; energized or fatigued; obviously or when others were unaware; at the gym or in my closet; when I succeeded or when I failed short; from the start of the day to the closing—_I prayed!_

2)   Throughout the day, I _'purposefully'_ focused and _'intentionally'_ planned to be a good steward over my spirit man, my temple and my gifts. Whereas, the book provides extensive details relative to each of these areas; below you will find a synopsis sufficient to propel you forward. It was apparent to me that I was on assignment as God's Agent, Attendant and Administrator of my Spirit man, my temple and the gifts He had gifted to me.

My life changed, things begin to happen on a new level. I was inspired to higher heights, my creativity was off the chain, my tolerance of others insults or immaturity was with ease, and my strength was amazing, even to me! And, the results were quite evident to those around me. RULE#4—I MUST fight knowing that I have already won

b)   Attendant of My temple} The book mentions several areas that are important to consider for proper caring of your temple. This *Journal* will only cover two of those.

1. Nutrition is extremely important whether you are on a fast or not. The condition of your physical health is greatly dependent upon what you put into your body—the temple! Of course, during the liquid fast my main focus was to be certain that I was getting essential nutrients from my liquids that I would ordinarily receive from solid foods. Since the fast, as I elaborate in detail in the book, I have a renewed perspective of food and its God created purpose

for my life! Gluttony, hoarding, recreational or event eating and so forth is no longer a part of my life—food does not control my life! In other words, *Food is NOT the boss of me!* I have seriously modified what, why and how I eat. Food is a *resource* for my physical wellbeing; no longer do I utilize it as a <u>source</u> for spiritual, emotional or mental fulfillment!

For the sake of those that have not read the book, my simplest suggestion is to encourage you to inquire of your healthcare provider or a certified nutritionist in this regard. Ask for their recommendation for the best diet plan/caloric intake to accommodate your individual needs!

2. Right alongside of nutrition is exercise—in fact, I call them the perfect partners! Exercise during my fast was limited because of my low caloric intake. I am a walker; I love to power walk—especially outside, weather permitting! In addition, I enjoy frequent visits to my local gym.

When I am not fasting, I try to work out at the gym at least 2-4 times per week. However, during the 40 day liquid fast, I had to forego strenuous exercise routines and be diligent to my leisurely walk either outside or on the treadmill. Regardless of what you do, exercise is a requirement! *Yes, my friend, we must get moving!*

c)   My gifts}   Every individual has unique gifting and has been blessed with their gifts to add value to ourselves and others. I clearly understood that God had gifted me in certain areas for the promoting of His Kingdom agenda and the benefit of others. (Review Ephesians 4:11-16 and 1 Corinthians 12:4-7)

During my 40 day fast, I received greater clarity; I was responsible for utilizing my gifts—being a good steward on a *daily* basis! Prior to the fast, I would casually use my gifts as the opportunity presented itself.   As I pressed closer to God, I embraced that stewardship of my gifts is a requirement and a responsibility. Not optional for use on occasions when I felt like it or when it was convenient. The matter was clear that He would require an account of how I used my gifts.[3] Furthermore, when I used my gifts to serve others, I brought God joy and I was personally fulfilled; being less focused on my challenges and needs.[4]

3)   Journaling is a great way to capture history in the making and to make notes relative to eventful utilization of your gifts on a daily basis. Take a few minutes to write down the highlights and significant occurrences of your day. You will be surprised of the impact, when a while later you reflect back on the very words that you have written. Your own words will be a wonderful source of encouragement, inspiration and energy to strengthen you to continue moving forward!

4)   At the end of each day I added a sealant—view this as your closing prayer! Simply thanking and praising God for providing you the strength to get through the day! Additionally, processing and examining before God the transactions that occurred throughout the day was vital to my success. Reflecting, repenting, and *listening* carefully to Him for further instructions or adjustments on my course operated as an accountability tool.

Our Loving Father is here and present! You can do this through the strength that He will provide you, as you become intimate with Him![5] He is your Champion—

---

[3] Luke 16:1-2/Romans 14:12
[4] Philippians 2:1-4
[5] Philippians 4:13

call upon Him and He will answer and show you great and mighty things that you know not of.[6]

Ok, my friend, you are on! *Let's get busy living* and operating in the quality life that God has predestined for each of His children! I am committed to praying for your success in Him! PLEASE keep me posted as you progress!

God has a plan...

and <u>YOU</u> are a part of it!

---

[6] Jeremiah 33:3

REVELATION

RULE NO. 1:

I **MUST** GET AN ELEVATED PERSPECTIVE OF WHOSE I AM AND WHO I AM IN HIM

Then God said, "Let Us make man in Our image, according to Our likeness.
They will <u>rule</u> the fish of the sea, the birds of the sky, the animals, all the earth, and the creatures that crawl on the earth."
So God created man in His own image; He created him in the image of God; He created them male and female.
God blessed them, and God said to them, "Be fruitful, multiply, fill the earth, and subdue it. <u>Rule</u> the fish of the sea, the birds of the sky, and every creature that crawls on the earth."
Genesis 1:26-28 (emphasis applied)

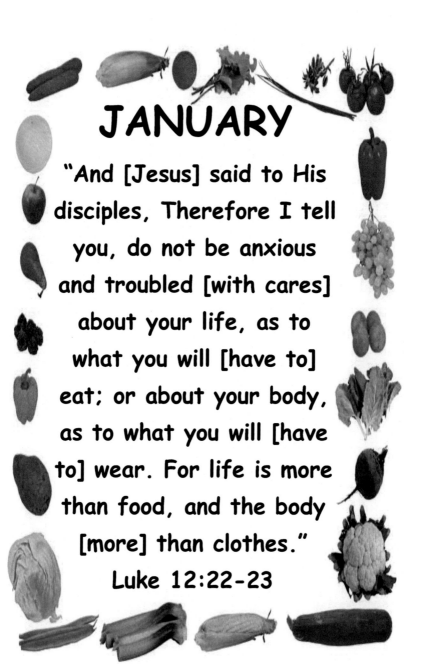

JANUARY

"And [Jesus] said to His disciples, Therefore I tell you, do not be anxious and troubled [with cares] about your life, as to what you will [have to] eat; or about your body, as to what you will [have to] wear. For life is more than food, and the body [more] than clothes."

Luke 12:22-23

January 1, _____ Day Start _____ End _____

My Prayer Focus _____

_____

Steward of My Spirit Man _____

_____

Steward of My Temple _____

_____

Steward of My Gifts _____

_____

Today I R.U.L.E. over My Life through:

Revelation	
Understanding	
Love	
Empowerment	

Exercise	
Nutrition	
Journal Notes	
Sealant	

You are precious in My sight and honored...Isaiah 43:4

January 2, _____ Day Start _____ End _____

My Prayer Focus _____

_____

Steward of My Spirit Man _____

_____

Steward of My Temple _____

_____

Steward of My Gifts _____

_____

Today I R.U.L.E. over My Life through:

Revelation	
Understanding	
Love	
Empowerment	

Exercise	
Nutrition	
Journal Notes	
Sealant	

January 3, _____ Day Start _____ End _____

My Prayer Focus _____

_____

Steward of My Spirit Man _____

_____

Steward of My Temple _____

_____

Steward of My Gifts _____

_____

Today I R.U.L.E. over My Life through:

Revelation	
Understanding	
Love	
Empowerment	

Exercise	
Nutrition	
Journal Notes	
Sealant	

Yet amid all these things we are more than conqueror and gain a surpassing victory through Him Who loved us Romans 8:37

January 4, _____ Day Start _____ End _____

My Prayer Focus _____

_____

Steward of My Spirit Man _____

_____

Steward of My Temple _____

_____

Steward of My Gifts _____

_____

Today I R.U.L.E. over My Life through:

Revelation	
Understanding	
Love	
Empowerment	

Exercise	
Nutrition	
Journal Notes	
Sealant	

January 5, _____ Day Start _____ End _____

My Prayer Focus _____

_____

Steward of My Spirit Man _____

_____

Steward of My Temple _____

_____

Steward of My Gifts _____

_____

Today I R.U.L.E. over My Life through:

Revelation	
Understanding	
Love	
Empowerment	

Exercise	
Nutrition	
Journal Notes	
Sealant	

Who has blessed us in Christ with every spiritual (given by the Holy Spirit) blessing in the heavenly realm...Ephesians 1:3

January 6, _____ Day Start _____ End _____

My Prayer Focus _____

_____

Steward of My Spirit Man _____

_____

Steward of My Temple _____

_____

Steward of My Gifts _____

_____

Today I R.U.L.E. over My Life through:

Revelation	
Understanding	
Love	
Empowerment	

Exercise	
Nutrition	
Journal Notes	
Sealant	

January 7, _____ Day Start _____ End _____

My Prayer Focus _____

_____

Steward of My Spirit Man _____

_____

Steward of My Temple _____

_____

Steward of My Gifts _____

_____

Today I R.U.L.E. over My Life through:

Revelation	
Understanding	
Love	
Empowerment	

Exercise	
Nutrition	
Journal Notes	
Sealant	

And you are in Him, made full and having come to fullness of life. Colossians 2:10

January 8, _____ Day Start _____ End _____

My Prayer Focus _____

_____

Steward of My Spirit Man _____

_____

Steward of My Temple _____

_____

Steward of My Gifts _____

_____

Today I R.U.L.E. over My Life through:

Revelation	
Understanding	
Love	
Empowerment	

Exercise	
Nutrition	
Journal Notes	
Sealant	

You are the light of the world. A city set on a hill cannot hidden. Matthew 5:14

January 9, _____   Day Start _____   End _____

My Prayer Focus _____

_____

Steward of My Spirit Man _____

_____

Steward of My Temple _____

_____

Steward of My Gifts _____

_____

Today I R.U.L.E. over My Life through:

Revelation	
Understanding	
Love	
Empowerment	

Exercise	
Nutrition	
Journal Notes	
Sealant	

To [you then] all God's beloved ones in Rome called to be saints and designated for a consecrated life. Romans 1:7

January 10,_____ Day Start _____ End _____

My Prayer Focus _____

_____

Steward of My Spirit Man _____

_____

Steward of My Temple _____

_____

Steward of My Gifts _____

_____

Today I R.U.L.E. over My Life through:

Revelation	
Understanding	
Love	
Empowerment	

Exercise	
Nutrition	
Journal Notes	
Sealant	

January 11,_____ Day Start _____ End _____

My Prayer Focus _____

_____

Steward of My Spirit Man _____

_____

Steward of My Temple _____

_____

Steward of My Gifts _____

_____

Today I R.U.L.E. over My Life through:

Revelation	
Understanding	
Love	
Empowerment	

Exercise	
Nutrition	
Journal Notes	
Sealant	

It is no longer I who live, but Christ (the Messiah) lives in me. Galatians 2:20

January 12,_____ Day Start _____ End _____

My Prayer Focus _____

_____

Steward of My Spirit Man _____

_____

Steward of My Temple _____

_____

Steward of My Gifts _____

_____

Today I R.U.L.E. over My Life through:

Revelation	
Understanding	
Love	
Empowerment	

Exercise	
Nutrition	
Journal Notes	
Sealant	

I live by faith in (by adherence to and reliance on and complete trust in) the Son of God. Galatians 2:20

January 13,_____ Day Start _____ End _____

My Prayer Focus _____

_____

Steward of My Spirit Man _____

_____

Steward of My Temple _____

_____

Steward of My Gifts _____

_____

Today I R.U.L.E. over My Life through:

Revelation	
Understanding	
Love	
Empowerment	

Exercise	
Nutrition	
Journal Notes	
Sealant	

He has clothed me with the garments of salvation; He has covered me with the robe of righteousness. Isaiah 61:10

January 14,_____ Day Start _____ End _____

My Prayer Focus _____

_____

Steward of My Spirit Man _____

_____

Steward of My Temple _____

_____

Steward of My Gifts _____

_____

Today I R.U.L.E. over My Life through:

Revelation	
Understanding	
Love	
Empowerment	

Exercise	
Nutrition	
Journal Notes	
Sealant	

January 15,_____ Day Start _____ End _____

My Prayer Focus _____

_____

Steward of My Spirit Man _____

_____

Steward of My Temple _____

_____

Steward of My Gifts _____

_____

Today I R.U.L.E. over My Life through:

Revelation	
Understanding	
Love	
Empowerment	

Exercise	
Nutrition	
Journal Notes	
Sealant	

January 16,_____ Day Start _____ End _____

My Prayer Focus _____

_____

Steward of My Spirit Man _____

_____

Steward of My Temple _____

_____

Steward of My Gifts _____

_____

Today I R.U.L.E. over My Life through:

Revelation	
Understanding	
Love	
Empowerment	

Exercise	
Nutrition	
Journal Notes	
Sealant	

If you will obey My voice in truth and keep My covenant, then you shall be My own peculiar possession and treasure. Exodus 19:5

January 17,_____ Day Start _____ End _____

My Prayer Focus _____

_____

Steward of My Spirit Man _____

_____

Steward of My Temple _____

_____

Steward of My Gifts _____

_____

Today I R.U.L.E. over My Life through:

Revelation	
Understanding	
Love	
Empowerment	

Exercise	
Nutrition	
Journal Notes	
Sealant	

January 18,_____ Day Start _____ End _____

My Prayer Focus _____

_____

Steward of My Spirit Man _____

_____

Steward of My Temple _____

_____

Steward of My Gifts _____

_____

Today I R.U.L.E. over My Life through:

Revelation	
Understanding	
Love	
Empowerment	

Exercise	
Nutrition	
Journal Notes	
Sealant	

January 19,_____ Day Start _____ End _____

My Prayer Focus _____

_____

Steward of My Spirit Man _____

_____

Steward of My Temple _____

_____

Steward of My Gifts _____

_____

Today I R.U.L.E. over My Life through:

Revelation	
Understanding	
Love	
Empowerment	

Exercise	
Nutrition	
Journal Notes	
Sealant	

For whatever is born of God is victorious over the world. 1 John 5:4

January 20,_____ Day Start _____ End _____

My Prayer Focus _____

_____

Steward of My Spirit Man _____

_____

Steward of My Temple _____

_____

Steward of My Gifts _____

_____

Today I R.U.L.E. over My Life through:

Revelation	
Understanding	
Love	
Empowerment	

Exercise		
Nutrition		
Journal Notes		
Sealant		

You must know (recognize) that you were redeemed (ransomed) from the useless (fruitless) way of living. 1 Peter 1:18

January 21,_____ Day Start _____ End _____

My Prayer Focus _____

_____

Steward of My Spirit Man _____

_____

Steward of My Temple _____

_____

Steward of My Gifts _____

_____

Today I R.U.L.E. over My Life through:

Revelation	
Understanding	
Love	
Empowerment	

Exercise	
Nutrition	
Journal Notes	
Sealant	

I pray that you may prosper in every way and [that your body] may keep well. 3 John 2

January 22,_____ Day Start _____ End _____

My Prayer Focus _____

_____

Steward of My Spirit Man _____

_____

Steward of My Temple _____

_____

Steward of My Gifts _____

_____

Today I R.U.L.E. over My Life through:

Revelation	
Understanding	
Love	
Empowerment	

Exercise	
Nutrition	
Journal Notes	
Sealant	

January 23,_____ Day Start _____ End _____

My Prayer Focus _____

_____

Steward of My Spirit Man _____

_____

Steward of My Temple _____

_____

Steward of My Gifts _____

_____

Today I R.U.L.E. over My Life through:

Revelation	
Understanding	
Love	
Empowerment	

Exercise	
Nutrition	
Journal Notes	
Sealant	

Not in your own strength, for it is God Who is all the while effectually at work in you. Philippians 2:13

January 24,_____ Day Start _____ End _____

My Prayer Focus _____

_____

Steward of My Spirit Man _____

_____

Steward of My Temple _____

_____

Steward of My Gifts _____

_____

Today I R.U.L.E. over My Life through:

Revelation	
Understanding	
Love	
Empowerment	

Exercise	
Nutrition	
Journal Notes	
Sealant	

January 25,_____ Day Start _____ End _____

My Prayer Focus _____

_____

Steward of My Spirit Man _____

_____

Steward of My Temple _____

_____

Steward of My Gifts _____

_____

Today I R.U.L.E. over My Life through:

Revelation	
Understanding	
Love	
Empowerment	

Exercise	
Nutrition	
Journal Notes	
Sealant	

Your word is a lamp to my feet and a light to my path. Psalm 119:105

January 26,_____ Day Start _____ End _____

My Prayer Focus _____

_____

Steward of My Spirit Man _____

_____

Steward of My Temple _____

_____

Steward of My Gifts _____

_____

Today I R.U.L.E. over My Life through:

Revelation	
Understanding	
Love	
Empowerment	

Exercise	
Nutrition	
Journal Notes	
Sealant	

You, through Your commandments, make me wiser than my enemies. Psalm 119:98

January 27,_____ Day Start _____ End _____

My Prayer Focus _____

_____

Steward of My Spirit Man _____

_____

Steward of My Temple _____

_____

Steward of My Gifts _____

_____

Today I R.U.L.E. over My Life through:

Revelation	
Understanding	
Love	
Empowerment	

Exercise	
Nutrition	
Journal Notes	
Sealant	

Get Wisdom (skilful and godly Wisdom)...wisdom is the principal thing...get understanding. Proverbs 4:7

January 28,_____ Day Start _____ End _____

My Prayer Focus _____

_____

Steward of My Spirit Man _____

_____

Steward of My Temple _____

_____

Steward of My Gifts _____

_____

Today I R.U.L.E. over My Life through:

Revelation	
Understanding	
Love	
Empowerment	

Exercise	
Nutrition	
Journal Notes	
Sealant	

January 29,_____ Day Start _____ End _____

My Prayer Focus _____

_____

Steward of My Spirit Man _____

_____

Steward of My Temple _____

_____

Steward of My Gifts _____

_____

Today I R.U.L.E. over My Life through:

Revelation	
Understanding	
Love	
Empowerment	

Exercise	
Nutrition	
Journal Notes	
Sealant	

For the Lord your God is bringing you into a good land. Deuteronomy 8:7

January 30,_____ Day Start _____ End _____

My Prayer Focus _____

_____

Steward of My Spirit Man _____

_____

Steward of My Temple _____

_____

Steward of My Gifts _____

_____

Today I R.U.L.E. over My Life through:

Revelation	
Understanding	
Love	
Empowerment	

Exercise	
Nutrition	
Journal Notes	
Sealant	

January 31,_____ Day Start _____ End _____

My Prayer Focus _____

_____

Steward of My Spirit Man _____

_____

Steward of My Temple _____

_____

Steward of My Gifts _____

_____

Today I R.U.L.E. over My Life through:

Revelation	
Understanding	
Love	
Empowerment	

Exercise	
Nutrition	
Journal Notes	
Sealant	

For in Him we live and move and have our being...some of your [own] poets have said, for we are also His offspring. Acts 17:28

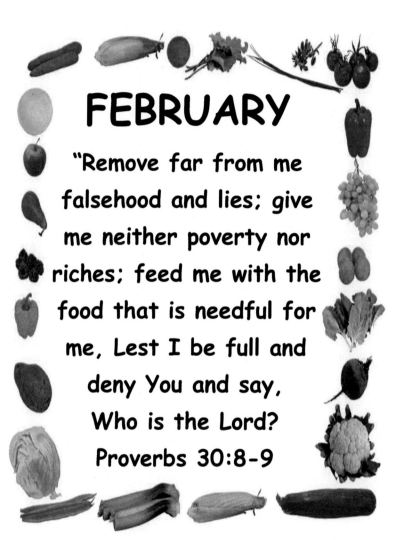

FEBRUARY

"Remove far from me falsehood and lies; give me neither poverty nor riches; feed me with the food that is needful for me, Lest I be full and deny You and say, Who is the Lord? Proverbs 30:8-9

February 1, _____ Day Start _____ End _____

My Prayer Focus _____

_____

Steward of My Spirit Man _____

_____

Steward of My Temple _____

_____

Steward of My Gifts _____

_____

Today I R.U.L.E. over My Life through:

Revelation	
Understanding	
Love	
Empowerment	

Exercise	
Nutrition	
Journal Notes	
Sealant	

February 2, _____ Day Start _____ End _____

My Prayer Focus _____

_____

Steward of My Spirit Man _____

_____

Steward of My Temple _____

_____

Steward of My Gifts _____

_____

Today I R.U.L.E. over My Life through:

Revelation	
Understanding	
Love	
Empowerment	

Exercise	
Nutrition	
Journal Notes	
Sealant	

Be transformed (changed) by the [entire] renewal of your mind [by its new ideals and its new attitude. Romans 12:2

February 3, _____ Day Start _____ End _____

My Prayer Focus _____

_____

Steward of My Spirit Man _____

_____

Steward of My Temple _____

_____

Steward of My Gifts _____

_____

Today I R.U.L.E. over My Life through:

Revelation	
Understanding	
Love	
Empowerment	

Exercise	
Nutrition	
Journal Notes	
Sealant	

February 4, _____ Day Start _____ End _____

My Prayer Focus _____

_____

Steward of My Spirit Man _____

_____

Steward of My Temple _____

_____

Steward of My Gifts _____

_____

Today I R.U.L.E. over My Life through:

Revelation	
Understanding	
Love	
Empowerment	

Exercise	
Nutrition	
Journal Notes	
Sealant	

He has a different spirit and has followed Me fully. Numbers 14:24

February 5, _____ Day Start _____ End _____

My Prayer Focus _____

_____

Steward of My Spirit Man _____

_____

Steward of My Temple _____

_____

Steward of My Gifts _____

_____

Today I R.U.L.E. over My Life through:

Revelation	
Understanding	
Love	
Empowerment	

Exercise	
Nutrition	
Journal Notes	
Sealant	

Choose for yourselves this day whom you will serve. Joshua 24:15

February 6, _____ Day Start _____ End _____

My Prayer Focus _____

_____

Steward of My Spirit Man _____

_____

Steward of My Temple _____

_____

Steward of My Gifts _____

_____

Today I R.U.L.E. over My Life through:

Revelation	
Understanding	
Love	
Empowerment	

Exercise	
Nutrition	
Journal Notes	
Sealant	

All that you say to me I will do. Ruth 3:5

February 7, _____ Day Start _____ End _____

My Prayer Focus _____

_____

Steward of My Spirit Man _____

_____

Steward of My Temple _____

_____

Steward of My Gifts _____

_____

Today I R.U.L.E. over My Life through:

Revelation	
Understanding	
Love	
Empowerment	

Exercise	
Nutrition	
Journal Notes	
Sealant	

February 8, _____ Day Start _____ End _____

My Prayer Focus _____

_____

Steward of My Spirit Man _____

_____

Steward of My Temple _____

_____

Steward of My Gifts _____

_____

Today I R.U.L.E. over My Life through:

Revelation	
Understanding	
Love	
Empowerment	

Exercise	
Nutrition	
Journal Notes	
Sealant	

February 9, _____ Day Start _____ End _____

My Prayer Focus _____

_____

Steward of My Spirit Man _____

_____

Steward of My Temple _____

_____

Steward of My Gifts _____

_____

Today I R.U.L.E. over My Life through:

Revelation	
Understanding	
Love	
Empowerment	

Exercise	
Nutrition	
Journal Notes	
Sealant	

You will guard him and keep him in perfect and constant peace whose mind is stayed on You. Isaiah 26:3

February 10,_____ Day Start _____ End _____

My Prayer Focus _____

_____

Steward of My Spirit Man _____

_____

Steward of My Temple _____

_____

Steward of My Gifts _____

_____

Today I R.U.L.E. over My Life through:

Revelation	
Understanding	
Love	
Empowerment	

Exercise	
Nutrition	
Journal Notes	
Sealant	

Because he commits himself to You, leans on You, and hopes confidently in You. Isaiah 26:3

February 11,_____ Day Start _____ End _____

My Prayer Focus _____

_____

Steward of My Spirit Man _____

_____

Steward of My Temple _____

_____

Steward of My Gifts _____

_____

Today I R.U.L.E. over My Life through:

Revelation	
Understanding	
Love	
Empowerment	

Exercise	
Nutrition	
Journal Notes	
Sealant	

I have told you these things, so that in Me you may have [perfect] peace and confidence. John 16:33

February 12,_____ Day Start _____ End _____

My Prayer Focus _____

_____

Steward of My Spirit Man _____

_____

Steward of My Temple _____

_____

Steward of My Gifts _____

_____

Today I R.U.L.E. over My Life through:

Revelation	
Understanding	
Love	
Empowerment	

Exercise	
Nutrition	
Journal Notes	
Sealant	

For I have overcome the world. [I have deprived it of power to harm you and have conquered it for you.] John 16:33

February 13,_____ Day Start _____ End _____

My Prayer Focus _____

_____

Steward of My Spirit Man _____

_____

Steward of My Temple _____

_____

Steward of My Gifts _____

_____

Today I R.U.L.E. over My Life through:

Revelation	
Understanding	
Love	
Empowerment	

Exercise	
Nutrition	
Journal Notes	
Sealant	

For God so greatly loved and dearly prized the world that He [even] gave up His only begotten ([a]unique) Son. John 3:16

February 14,_____ Day Start _____ End _____

My Prayer Focus _____

_____

Steward of My Spirit Man _____

_____

Steward of My Temple _____

_____

Steward of My Gifts _____

_____

Today I R.U.L.E. over My Life through:

Revelation	
Understanding	
Love	
Empowerment	

Exercise	
Nutrition	
Journal Notes	
Sealant	

February 15,_____ Day Start _____ End _____

My Prayer Focus _____

_____

Steward of My Spirit Man _____

_____

Steward of My Temple _____

_____

Steward of My Gifts _____

_____

Today I R.U.L.E. over My Life through:

Revelation	
Understanding	
Love	
Empowerment	

Exercise	
Nutrition	
Journal Notes	
Sealant	

February 16,_____ Day Start _____ End _____

My Prayer Focus _____

_____

Steward of My Spirit Man _____

_____

Steward of My Temple _____

_____

Steward of My Gifts _____

_____

Today I R.U.L.E. over My Life through:

Revelation	
Understanding	
Love	
Empowerment	

Exercise	
Nutrition	
Journal Notes	
Sealant	

And endurance (fortitude) develops maturity of character (approved faith and tried integrity). Romans 5:4

February 17,_____ Day Start _____ End _____

My Prayer Focus _____

_____

Steward of My Spirit Man _____

_____

Steward of My Temple _____

_____

Steward of My Gifts _____

_____

Today I R.U.L.E. over My Life through:

Revelation	
Understanding	
Love	
Empowerment	

Exercise	
Nutrition	
Journal Notes	
Sealant	

It is good that one should hope in and wait quietly for the salvation (the safety and ease) of the Lord. Lamentations 3:26

February 18,_____ Day Start _____ End _____

My Prayer Focus _____

_____

Steward of My Spirit Man _____

_____

Steward of My Temple _____

_____

Steward of My Gifts _____

_____

Today I R.U.L.E. over My Life through:

Revelation	
Understanding	
Love	
Empowerment	

Exercise	
Nutrition	
Journal Notes	
Sealant	

Christ within and among you, the Hope of [realizing the] glory. Colossians 1:27

February 19,____ Day Start ____ End ____

My Prayer Focus _____

_____

Steward of My Spirit Man _____

_____

Steward of My Temple _____

_____

Steward of My Gifts _____

_____

Today I R.U.L.E. over My Life through:

Revelation	
Understanding	
Love	
Empowerment	

Exercise	
Nutrition	
Journal Notes	
Sealant	

I hoped in Your word. Psalm 119:147

February 20,____ Day Start _____ End _____

My Prayer Focus _____

_____

Steward of My Spirit Man _____

_____

Steward of My Temple _____

_____

Steward of My Gifts _____

_____

Today I R.U.L.E. over My Life through:

Revelation	
Understanding	
Love	
Empowerment	

Exercise	
Nutrition	
Journal Notes	
Sealant	

And God said, Let there be light; and there was light. Genesis 1:3

February 21,_____ Day Start _____ End _____

My Prayer Focus _____

_____

Steward of My Spirit Man _____

_____

Steward of My Temple _____

_____

Steward of My Gifts _____

_____

Today I R.U.L.E. over My Life through:

Revelation	
Understanding	
Love	
Empowerment	

Exercise	
Nutrition	
Journal Notes	
Sealant	

You ... decide and decree a thing... it shall be established for you...the **light** [of God's favor] shall **shine** upon your ways. Job 22:28

February 22,_____Day Start _____ End _____

My Prayer Focus _____

_____

Steward of My Spirit Man _____

_____

Steward of My Temple _____

_____

Steward of My Gifts _____

_____

Today I R.U.L.E. over My Life through:

Revelation	
Understanding	
Love	
Empowerment	

Exercise	
Nutrition	
Journal Notes	
Sealant	

February 23,_____ Day Start _____ End _____

My Prayer Focus _____

_____

Steward of My Spirit Man _____

_____

Steward of My Temple _____

_____

Steward of My Gifts _____

_____

Today I R.U.L.E. over My Life through:

Revelation	
Understanding	
Love	
Empowerment	

Exercise	
Nutrition	
Journal Notes	
Sealant	

Now you are light in the Lord; walk as children of Light. Ephesians 5:8

February 24,_____ Day Start _____ End _____

My Prayer Focus _____

_____

Steward of My Spirit Man _____

_____

Steward of My Temple _____

_____

Steward of My Gifts _____

_____

Today I R.U.L.E. over My Life through:

Revelation	
Understanding	
Love	
Empowerment	

Exercise		
Nutrition		
Journal Notes		
Sealant		

February 25,_____ Day Start _____ End _____

My Prayer Focus _____

_____

Steward of My Spirit Man _____

_____

Steward of My Temple _____

_____

Steward of My Gifts _____

_____

Today I R.U.L.E. over My Life through:

Revelation	
Understanding	
Love	
Empowerment	

Exercise	
Nutrition	
Journal Notes	
Sealant	

February 26,_____ Day Start _____ End _____

My Prayer Focus _____

_____

Steward of My Spirit Man _____

_____

Steward of My Temple _____

_____

Steward of My Gifts _____

_____

Today I R.U.L.E. over My Life through:

Revelation	
Understanding	
Love	
Empowerment	

Exercise	
Nutrition	
Journal Notes	
Sealant	

February 27,_____ Day Start _____ End _____

My Prayer Focus _____

_____

Steward of My Spirit Man _____

_____

Steward of My Temple _____

_____

Steward of My Gifts _____

_____

Today I R.U.L.E. over My Life through:

Revelation	
Understanding	
Love	
Empowerment	

Exercise	
Nutrition	
Journal Notes	
Sealant	

What therefore God has joined **together**, let not man **put** asunder (separate). Matthew 19:6

February 28,_____ Day Start _____ End _____

My Prayer Focus _____

_____

Steward of My Spirit Man _____

_____

Steward of My Temple _____

_____

Steward of My Gifts _____

_____

Today I R.U.L.E. over My Life through:

Revelation	
Understanding	
Love	
Empowerment	

Exercise	
Nutrition	
Journal Notes	
Sealant	

February 29,_____ Day Start _____ End _____

My Prayer Focus _____

_____

Steward of My Spirit Man _____

_____

Steward of My Temple _____

_____

Steward of My Gifts _____

_____

Today I R.U.L.E. over My Life through:

Revelation	
Understanding	
Love	
Empowerment	

Exercise	
Nutrition	
Journal Notes	
Sealant	

I in them and You in Me, in order that they may become one and perfectly united, that the world may know. John 17:23

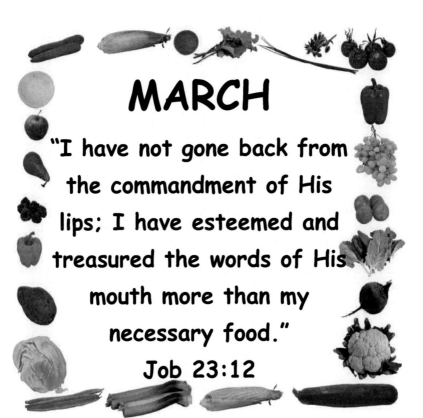

MARCH

"I have not gone back from the commandment of His lips; I have esteemed and treasured the words of His mouth more than my necessary food."

Job 23:12

March 1, _____ Day Start _____ End _____

My Prayer Focus _____

_____

Steward of My Spirit Man _____

_____

Steward of My Temple _____

_____

Steward of My Gifts _____

_____

Today I R.U.L.E. over My Life through:

Revelation	
Understanding	
Love	
Empowerment	

Exercise		
Nutrition		
Journal Notes		
Sealant		

March 2, _____ Day Start _____ End _____

My Prayer Focus _____

_____

Steward of My Spirit Man _____

_____

Steward of My Temple _____

_____

Steward of My Gifts _____

_____

Today I R.U.L.E. over My Life through:

Revelation	
Understanding	
Love	
Empowerment	

Exercise	
Nutrition	
Journal Notes	
Sealant	

Let not him who eats despise him who does not eat, and let not him who does not eat judge him who eats...Romans 14:3 NKJV

March 3, _____ Day Start _____ End _____

My Prayer Focus _____
_____

Steward of My Spirit Man _____
_____

Steward of My Temple _____
_____

Steward of My Gifts _____
_____

Today I R.U.L.E. over My Life through:

Revelation	
Understanding	
Love	
Empowerment	

Exercise	
Nutrition	
Journal Notes	
Sealant	

For I am already about to be sacrificed [my life is about to be poured out as a drink offering]...2 Timothy 4:6

March 4, _____ Day Start _____ End _____

My Prayer Focus _____

_____

Steward of My Spirit Man _____

_____

Steward of My Temple _____

_____

Steward of My Gifts _____

_____

Today I R.U.L.E. over My Life through:

Revelation	
Understanding	
Love	
Empowerment	

Exercise	
Nutrition	
Journal Notes	
Sealant	

He causes vegetation to grow for the cattle, and all that the earth produces for man to cultivate...Psalm 104:14

March 5, _____ Day Start ____ End ____

My Prayer Focus _____

_____

Steward of My Spirit Man _____

_____

Steward of My Temple _____

_____

Steward of My Gifts _____

_____

Today I R.U.L.E. over My Life through:

Revelation	
Understanding	
Love	
Empowerment	

Exercise	
Nutrition	
Journal Notes	
Sealant	

That he may bring forth food out of the earth...and bread to support, refresh, and strengthen man's heart. Psalm 104:14-15

March 6, _____ Day Start ____ End ____

My Prayer Focus _____

_____

Steward of My Spirit Man _____

_____

Steward of My Temple _____

_____

Steward of My Gifts _____

_____

Today I R.U.L.E. over My Life through:

Revelation	
Understanding	
Love	
Empowerment	

Exercise	
Nutrition	
Journal Notes	
Sealant	

March 7, _____ Day Start _____ End _____

My Prayer Focus _____

_____

Steward of My Spirit Man _____

_____

Steward of My Temple _____

_____

Steward of My Gifts _____

_____

Today I R.U.L.E. over My Life through:

Revelation	
Understanding	
Love	
Empowerment	

Exercise	
Nutrition	
Journal Notes	
Sealant	

Much food is in the tilled land of the poor, but there are those who are destroyed because of injustice. Proverbs 13:23

March 8, _____ Day Start _____ End _____

My Prayer Focus _____

_____

Steward of My Spirit Man _____

_____

Steward of My Temple _____

_____

Steward of My Gifts _____

_____

Today I R.U.L.E. over My Life through:

Revelation	
Understanding	
Love	
Empowerment	

Exercise	
Nutrition	
Journal Notes	
Sealant	

Happy (blessed, fortunate, enviable) is he who has the God of...Jacob for his help, whose hope is in the Lord. Psalm 146:5

March 9, _____ Day Start _____ End _____

My Prayer Focus _____

_____

Steward of My Spirit Man _____

_____

Steward of My Temple _____

_____

Steward of My Gifts _____

_____

Today I R.U.L.E. over My Life through:

Revelation	
Understanding	
Love	
Empowerment	

Exercise	
Nutrition	
Journal Notes	
Sealant	

Who executes justice for the oppressed, Who gives food to the hungry. The Lord sets free the prisoners. Psalm s 146:7

March 10, _____ Day Start _____ End _____

My Prayer Focus _____

_____

Steward of My Spirit Man _____

_____

Steward of My Temple _____

_____

Steward of My Gifts _____

_____

Today I R.U.L.E. over My Life through:

Revelation	
Understanding	
Love	
Empowerment	

Exercise	
Nutrition	
Journal Notes	
Sealant	

March 11, _____ Day Start _____ End _____

My Prayer Focus _____

_____

Steward of My Spirit Man _____

_____

Steward of My Temple _____

_____

Steward of My Gifts _____

_____

Today I R.U.L.E. over My Life through:

Revelation	
Understanding	
Love	
Empowerment	

Exercise	
Nutrition	
Journal Notes	
Sealant	

If a brother or sister...lacks food for each day...without giving him the necessities for the body, what good does that do? James 2:16

March 12, _____ Day Start _____ End _____

My Prayer Focus _____

_____

Steward of My Spirit Man _____

_____

Steward of My Temple _____

_____

Steward of My Gifts _____

_____

Today I R.U.L.E. over My Life through:

Revelation	
Understanding	
Love	
Empowerment	

Exercise	
Nutrition	
Journal Notes	
Sealant	

When the sun is down, he shall be clean, and afterward may eat of the holy things, for they are his food. Leviticus 22:7

March 13, _____ Day Start ____ End ____

My Prayer Focus _____

_____

Steward of My Spirit Man _____

_____

Steward of My Temple _____

_____

Steward of My Gifts _____

_____

Today I R.U.L.E. over My Life through:

Revelation	
Understanding	
Love	
Empowerment	

Exercise	
Nutrition	
Journal Notes	
Sealant	

Who provides for the raven its prey when its young ones cry to God and wander about for lack of food? Job 38:41

March 14, _____ Day Start _____ End _____

My Prayer Focus _____

_____

Steward of My Spirit Man _____

_____

Steward of My Temple _____

_____

Steward of My Gifts _____

_____

Today I R.U.L.E. over My Life through:

Revelation	
Understanding	
Love	
Empowerment	

Exercise	
Nutrition	
Journal Notes	
Sealant	

March 15, _____ Day Start _____ End _____

My Prayer Focus _____

_____

Steward of My Spirit Man _____

_____

Steward of My Temple _____

_____

Steward of My Gifts _____

_____

Today I R.U.L.E. over My Life through:

Revelation	
Understanding	
Love	
Empowerment	

Exercise	
Nutrition	
Journal Notes	
Sealant	

And there will be goats milk enough for your food, for the food of your household... Proverbs 27:27

March 16, _____ Day Start _____ End _____

My Prayer Focus _____

_____

Steward of My Spirit Man _____

_____

Steward of My Temple _____

_____

Steward of My Gifts _____

_____

Today I R.U.L.E. over My Life through:

Revelation	
Understanding	
Love	
Empowerment	

Exercise	
Nutrition	
Journal Notes	
Sealant	

...but Mephibosheth, your master's son [grandson], shall eat always at my table. 2 Samuel 9:10

March 17, _____ Day Start _____ End _____

My Prayer Focus _____

_____

Steward of My Spirit Man _____

_____

Steward of My Temple _____

_____

Steward of My Gifts _____

_____

Today I R.U.L.E. over My Life through:

Revelation	
Understanding	
Love	
Empowerment	

Exercise	
Nutrition	
Journal Notes	
Sealant	

He executes justice for the fatherless and the widow, and loves the stranger...gives him food and clothing. Deuteronomy 10:18

March 18, _____ Day Start _____ End _____

My Prayer Focus _____

_____

Steward of My Spirit Man _____

_____

Steward of My Temple _____

_____

Steward of My Gifts _____

_____

Today I R.U.L.E. over My Life through:

Revelation	
Understanding	
Love	
Empowerment	

Exercise	
Nutrition	
Journal Notes	
Sealant	

March 19, _____ Day Start _____ End _____

My Prayer Focus _____

_____

Steward of My Spirit Man _____

_____

Steward of My Temple _____

_____

Steward of My Gifts _____

_____

Today I R.U.L.E. over My Life through:

Revelation	
Understanding	
Love	
Empowerment	

Exercise	
Nutrition	
Journal Notes	
Sealant	

He blessed Joseph, and said "God, before whom my fathers Abraham and Isaac walked...fed me all my life long." Genesis 48:15

March 20, _____ Day Start _____ End _____

My Prayer Focus _____

_____

Steward of My Spirit Man _____

_____

Steward of My Temple _____

_____

Steward of My Gifts _____

_____

Today I R.U.L.E. over My Life through:

Revelation	
Understanding	
Love	
Empowerment	

Exercise		
Nutrition		
Journal Notes		
Sealant		

March 21, _____ Day Start _____ End _____

My Prayer Focus _____

_____

Steward of My Spirit Man _____

_____

Steward of My Temple _____

_____

Steward of My Gifts _____

_____

Today I R.U.L.E. over My Life through:

Revelation	
Understanding	
Love	
Empowerment	

Exercise	
Nutrition	
Journal Notes	
Sealant	

I was hungry and you gave Me food; I was thirsty and you gave Me drink; I was a stranger and you took Me in. Matthew 25:35

March 22, _____ Day Start ____ End ____

My Prayer Focus _____

_____

Steward of My Spirit Man _____

_____

Steward of My Temple _____

_____

Steward of My Gifts _____

_____

Today I R.U.L.E. over My Life through:

Revelation	
Understanding	
Love	
Empowerment	

Exercise	
Nutrition	
Journal Notes	
Sealant	

Then the just and upright will answer Him, Lord, when did we see You hungry and gave You food? Matthew 25:35

March 23, _____ Day Start _____ End _____

My Prayer Focus _____

_____

Steward of My Spirit Man _____

_____

Steward of My Temple _____

_____

Steward of My Gifts _____

_____

Today I R.U.L.E. over My Life through:

Revelation	
Understanding	
Love	
Empowerment	

Exercise	
Nutrition	
Journal Notes	
Sealant	

March 24, _____ Day Start _____ End _____

My Prayer Focus _____

_____

Steward of My Spirit Man _____

_____

Steward of My Temple _____

_____

Steward of My Gifts _____

_____

Today I R.U.L.E. over My Life through:

Revelation	
Understanding	
Love	
Empowerment	

Exercise	
Nutrition	
Journal Notes	
Sealant	

I fed and shepherded the flock. Zechariah 11:7

March 25, _____ Day Start _____ End _____

My Prayer Focus _____

_____

Steward of My Spirit Man _____

_____

Steward of My Temple _____

_____

Steward of My Gifts _____

_____

Today I R.U.L.E. over My Life through:

Revelation	
Understanding	
Love	
Empowerment	

Exercise	
Nutrition	
Journal Notes	
Sealant	

And Esau said to Jacob, Feed me, I pray thee, with that same red pottage; for I am faint. Genesis 25:30 KJV

March 26, _____ Day Start _____ End _____

My Prayer Focus _____

_____

Steward of My Spirit Man _____

_____

Steward of My Temple _____

_____

Steward of My Gifts _____

_____

Today I R.U.L.E. over My Life through:

Revelation	
Understanding	
Love	
Empowerment	

Exercise	
Nutrition	
Journal Notes	
Sealant	

You have fed them with the bread of tears, and You have given them tears to drink in large measure. Psalm 80:5

March 27, _____ Day Start _____ End _____

My Prayer Focus _____

_____

Steward of My Spirit Man _____

_____

Steward of My Temple _____

_____

Steward of My Gifts _____

_____

Today I R.U.L.E. over My Life through:

Revelation	
Understanding	
Love	
Empowerment	

Exercise	
Nutrition	
Journal Notes	
Sealant	

These are spots in your feasts of charity, when they feast with you, feeding themselves without fear. Jude 12 KJV

March 28, _____ Day Start _____ End _____

My Prayer Focus _____

_____

Steward of My Spirit Man _____

_____

Steward of My Temple _____

_____

Steward of My Gifts _____

_____

Today I R.U.L.E. over My Life through:

Revelation	
Understanding	
Love	
Empowerment	

Exercise		
Nutrition		
Journal Notes		
Sealant		

The heart of him that hath understanding seeketh knowledge: but the mouth of fools feedeth on foolishness. Proverbs 15:14 KJV

March 29, _____ Day Start _____ End _____

My Prayer Focus _____

_____

Steward of My Spirit Man _____

_____

Steward of My Temple _____

_____

Steward of My Gifts _____

_____

Today I R.U.L.E. over My Life through:

Revelation	
Understanding	
Love	
Empowerment	

Exercise	
Nutrition	
Journal Notes	
Sealant	

Observe and consider the ravens; for they neither sow nor reap... God feeds them. Luke 12:24

March 30, _____ Day Start _____ End _____

My Prayer Focus _____

_____

Steward of My Spirit Man _____

_____

Steward of My Temple _____

_____

Steward of My Gifts _____

_____

Today I R.U.L.E. over My Life through:

Revelation	
Understanding	
Love	
Empowerment	

Exercise	
Nutrition	
Journal Notes	
Sealant	

March 31, _____ Day Start _____ End _____

My Prayer Focus _____

_____

Steward of My Spirit Man _____

_____

Steward of My Temple _____

_____

Steward of My Gifts _____

_____

Today I R.U.L.E. over My Life through:

Revelation	
Understanding	
Love	
Empowerment	

Exercise	
Nutrition	
Journal Notes	
Sealant	

For Israel has behaved stubbornly, like a stubborn heifer. How then should he expect to be fed and treated by the Lord? Hosea 4:16

UNDERSTANDING

RULE NO. 2:

EVERY TEMPTATION MUST SUBMIT TO MY AUTHORITY

*There hath no temptation
taken you but such as is common
to man: but God is faithful, who will
not suffer you to be tempted above that
ye are able; but will with the temptation also
make a way to escape, that ye may be able to
bear it.*
1 Corinthians 10:13

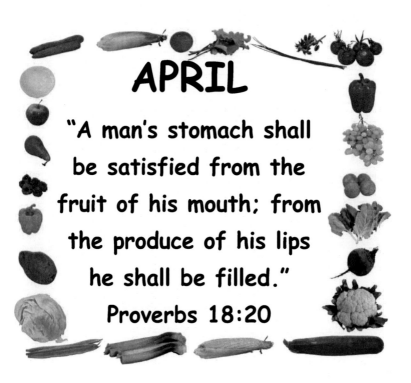

APRIL

"A man's stomach shall be satisfied from the fruit of his mouth; from the produce of his lips he shall be filled."

Proverbs 18:20

April 1, _____ Day Start _____ End _____

My Prayer Focus _____

_____

Steward of My Spirit Man _____

_____

Steward of My Temple _____

_____

Steward of My Gifts _____

_____

Today I R.U.L.E. over My Life through:

Revelation	
Understanding	
Love	
Empowerment	

Exercise	
Nutrition	
Journal Notes	
Sealant	

Truthful lips shall be established forever, but a lying tongue is [credited] but for a moment. Proverbs 12:19

April 2, _____ Day Start _____ End _____

My Prayer Focus _____

_____

Steward of My Spirit Man _____

_____

Steward of My Temple _____

_____

Steward of My Gifts _____

_____

Today I R.U.L.E. over My Life through:

Revelation	
Understanding	
Love	
Empowerment	

Exercise	
Nutrition	
Journal Notes	
Sealant	

Hannah was speaking in her heart; only her lips moved but her voice was not heard. 1 Samuel 1:13

April 3, _____ Day Start _____ End _____

My Prayer Focus _____

_____

Steward of My Spirit Man _____

_____

Steward of My Temple _____

_____

Steward of My Gifts _____

_____

Today I R.U.L.E. over My Life through:

Revelation	
Understanding	
Love	
Empowerment	

Exercise	
Nutrition	
Journal Notes	
Sealant	

O Lord, open my lips, and my mouth shall show forth Your praise. Psalm 51:15

April 4, _____ Day Start _____ End _____

My Prayer Focus _____

_____

Steward of My Spirit Man _____

_____

Steward of My Temple _____

_____

Steward of My Gifts _____

_____

Today I R.U.L.E. over My Life through:

Revelation	
Understanding	
Love	
Empowerment	

Exercise	
Nutrition	
Journal Notes	
Sealant	

The lips of the [uncompromisingly] righteous feed and guide many. Proverbs 10:21

April 5, _____ Day Start _____ End _____

My Prayer Focus _____

_____

Steward of My Spirit Man _____

_____

Steward of My Temple _____

_____

Steward of My Gifts _____

_____

Today I R.U.L.E. over My Life through:

Revelation	
Understanding	
Love	
Empowerment	

Exercise	
Nutrition	
Journal Notes	
Sealant	

April 6, _____ Day Start ____ End ____

My Prayer Focus _____

_____

Steward of My Spirit Man _____

_____

Steward of My Temple _____

_____

Steward of My Gifts _____

_____

Today I R.U.L.E. over My Life through:

Revelation	
Understanding	
Love	
Empowerment	

Exercise	
Nutrition	
Journal Notes	
Sealant	

April 7, _____ Day Start _____ End _____

My Prayer Focus _____

_____

Steward of My Spirit Man _____

_____

Steward of My Temple _____

_____

Steward of My Gifts _____

_____

Today I R.U.L.E. over My Life through:

Revelation	
Understanding	
Love	
Empowerment	

Exercise	
Nutrition	
Journal Notes	
Sealant	

The words of a wise man's mouth are gracious and win him favor, but the lips of a fool consume him. Ecclesiastes 10:12

April 8, _____ Day Start _____ End _____

My Prayer Focus _____

_____

Steward of My Spirit Man _____

_____

Steward of My Temple _____

_____

Steward of My Gifts _____

_____

Today I R.U.L.E. over My Life through:

Revelation	
Understanding	
Love	
Empowerment	

Exercise	
Nutrition	
Journal Notes	
Sealant	

April 9, _____ Day Start _____ End _____

My Prayer Focus _____

_____

Steward of My Spirit Man _____

_____

Steward of My Temple _____

_____

Steward of My Gifts _____

_____

Today I R.U.L.E. over My Life through:

Revelation	
Understanding	
Love	
Empowerment	

Exercise	
Nutrition	
Journal Notes	
Sealant	

And with it he touched my mouth and said, Behold, this has touched your lips; your iniquity and guilt are taken away...Isaiah 6:7

April 10, _____ Day Start _____ End _____

My Prayer Focus _____

_____

Steward of My Spirit Man _____

_____

Steward of My Temple _____

_____

Steward of My Gifts _____

_____

Today I R.U.L.E. over My Life through:

Revelation	
Understanding	
Love	
Empowerment	

Exercise	
Nutrition	
Journal Notes	
Sealant	

And your sin is completely atoned for and forgiven. Isaiah 6:7

April 11, _____ Day Start _____ End _____

My Prayer Focus _____

_____

Steward of My Spirit Man _____

_____

Steward of My Temple _____

_____

Steward of My Gifts _____

_____

Today I R.U.L.E. over My Life through:

Revelation	
Understanding	
Love	
Empowerment	

Exercise	
Nutrition	
Journal Notes	
Sealant	

In [spite of] all this, Job did not sin with his lips. Job 2:10

April 12, _____ Day Start _____ End _____

My Prayer Focus _____

_____

Steward of My Spirit Man _____

_____

Steward of My Temple _____

_____

Steward of My Gifts _____

_____

Today I R.U.L.E. over My Life through:

Revelation	
Understanding	
Love	
Empowerment	

Exercise		
Nutrition		
Journal Notes		
Sealant		

April 13, _____ Day Start _____ End _____

My Prayer Focus _____

_____

Steward of My Spirit Man _____

_____

Steward of My Temple _____

_____

Steward of My Gifts _____

_____

Today I R.U.L.E. over My Life through:

Revelation	
Understanding	
Love	
Empowerment	

Exercise	
Nutrition	
Journal Notes	
Sealant	

Let us constantly and at all times offer up to God a sacrifice of praise, which is the fruit of lips. Hebrews 13:15

April 14, _____ Day Start ____ End ____

My Prayer Focus _____

_____

Steward of My Spirit Man _____

_____

Steward of My Temple _____

_____

Steward of My Gifts _____

_____

Today I R.U.L.E. over My Life through:

Revelation	
Understanding	
Love	
Empowerment	

Exercise	
Nutrition	
Journal Notes	
Sealant	

For let him who wants to enjoy life and see good days ...keep his tongue free from evil and his lips from guile. 1 Peter 3:10

April 15, _____ Day Start _____ End _____

My Prayer Focus _____

_____

Steward of My Spirit Man _____

_____

Steward of My Temple _____

_____

Steward of My Gifts _____

_____

Today I R.U.L.E. over My Life through:

Revelation	
Understanding	
Love	
Empowerment	

Exercise	
Nutrition	
Journal Notes	
Sealant	

Behold, the children of Israel have not hearkened unto me...shall Pharaoh hear me, who am of uncircumcised lips? Exodus 6:12

April 16, _____ Day Start _____ End _____

My Prayer Focus _____

_____

Steward of My Spirit Man _____

_____

Steward of My Temple _____

_____

Steward of My Gifts _____

_____

Today I R.U.L.E. over My Life through:

Revelation	
Understanding	
Love	
Empowerment	

Exercise	
Nutrition	
Journal Notes	
Sealant	

To his neighbor each one speaks words without...truth; with flattering lips and double heart [deceitfully]. Psalm 12:2

April 17, _____ Day Start ____ End ____

My Prayer Focus _____

_____

Steward of My Spirit Man _____

_____

Steward of My Temple _____

_____

Steward of My Gifts _____

_____

Today I R.U.L.E. over My Life through:

Revelation	
Understanding	
Love	
Empowerment	

Exercise	
Nutrition	
Journal Notes	
Sealant	

April 18, _____ Day Start _____ End _____

My Prayer Focus _____

_____

Steward of My Spirit Man _____

_____

Steward of My Temple _____

_____

Steward of My Gifts _____

_____

Today I R.U.L.E. over My Life through:

Revelation	
Understanding	
Love	
Empowerment	

Exercise	
Nutrition	
Journal Notes	
Sealant	

Who have said, With our tongue will we prevail; our lips are our own: who is lord over us? Psalm 12:4 KJV

April 19, _____ Day Start _____ End _____

My Prayer Focus _____

_____

Steward of My Spirit Man _____

_____

Steward of My Temple _____

_____

Steward of My Gifts _____

_____

Today I R.U.L.E. over My Life through:

Revelation	
Understanding	
Love	
Empowerment	

Exercise	
Nutrition	
Journal Notes	
Sealant	

April 20, _____ Day Start _____ End _____

My Prayer Focus _____

_____

Steward of My Spirit Man _____

_____

Steward of My Temple _____

_____

Steward of My Gifts _____

_____

Today I R.U.L.E. over My Life through:

Revelation	
Understanding	
Love	
Empowerment	

Exercise	
Nutrition	
Journal Notes	
Sealant	

April 21, _____ Day Start ____ End ____

My Prayer Focus _____

_____

Steward of My Spirit Man _____

_____

Steward of My Temple _____

_____

Steward of My Gifts _____

_____

Today I R.U.L.E. over My Life through:

Revelation	
Understanding	
Love	
Empowerment	

Exercise	
Nutrition	
Journal Notes	
Sealant	

April 22, _____ Day Start _____ End _____

My Prayer Focus _____

_____

Steward of My Spirit Man _____

_____

Steward of My Temple _____

_____

Steward of My Gifts _____

_____

Today I R.U.L.E. over My Life through:

Revelation	
Understanding	
Love	
Empowerment	

Exercise	
Nutrition	
Journal Notes	
Sealant	

Because Your loving-kindness is better than life, my lips shall praise You. Psalm 63:3

April 23, _____ Day Start _____ End _____

My Prayer Focus _____

_____

Steward of My Spirit Man _____

_____

Steward of My Temple _____

_____

Steward of My Gifts _____

_____

Today I R.U.L.E. over My Life through:

Revelation	
Understanding	
Love	
Empowerment	

Exercise	
Nutrition	
Journal Notes	
Sealant	

My whole being shall be satisfied as with marrow and fatness; and my mouth shall praise You with joyful lips. Psalm 63:5

April 24, _____ Day Start _____ End _____

My Prayer Focus _____

_____

Steward of My Spirit Man _____

_____

Steward of My Temple _____

_____

Steward of My Gifts _____

_____

Today I R.U.L.E. over My Life through:

Revelation	
Understanding	
Love	
Empowerment	

Exercise	
Nutrition	
Journal Notes	
Sealant	

Behold, they belch out [insults] with their mouths; swords [of sarcasm, ridicule, slander, and lies] are in their lips...Psalm 59:7

April 25, _____ Day Start _____ End _____

My Prayer Focus _____

_____

Steward of My Spirit Man _____

_____

Steward of My Temple _____

_____

Steward of My Gifts _____

_____

Today I R.U.L.E. over My Life through:

Revelation	
Understanding	
Love	
Empowerment	

Exercise	
Nutrition	
Journal Notes	
Sealant	

April 26, _____ Day Start _____ End _____

My Prayer Focus _____

_____

Steward of My Spirit Man _____

_____

Steward of My Temple _____

_____

Steward of My Gifts _____

_____

Today I R.U.L.E. over My Life through:

Revelation	
Understanding	
Love	
Empowerment	

Exercise	
Nutrition	
Journal Notes	
Sealant	

April 27, _____ Day Start _____ End _____

My Prayer Focus _____

_____

Steward of My Spirit Man _____

_____

Steward of My Temple _____

_____

Steward of My Gifts _____

_____

Today I R.U.L.E. over My Life through:

Revelation	
Understanding	
Love	
Empowerment	

Exercise	
Nutrition	
Journal Notes	
Sealant	

I will make you a name and a praise among all the nations of the earth when I reverse your captivity. Zephaniah 3:20

April 28, _____ Day Start _____ End _____

My Prayer Focus _____

_____

Steward of My Spirit Man _____

_____

Steward of My Temple _____

_____

Steward of My Gifts _____

_____

Today I R.U.L.E. over My Life through:

Revelation	
Understanding	
Love	
Empowerment	

Exercise	
Nutrition	
Journal Notes	
Sealant	

You are fairer than the children of men; graciousness is poured upon Your lips; therefore God has blessed You forever. Psalm 45:2

April 29, _____ Day Start _____ End _____

My Prayer Focus _____

_____

Steward of My Spirit Man _____

_____

Steward of My Temple _____

_____

Steward of My Gifts _____

_____

Today I R.U.L.E. over My Life through:

Revelation	
Understanding	
Love	
Empowerment	

Exercise	
Nutrition	
Journal Notes	
Sealant	

April 30, _____ Day Start _____ End _____

My Prayer Focus _____

_____

Steward of My Spirit Man _____

_____

Steward of My Temple _____

_____

Steward of My Gifts _____

_____

Today I R.U.L.E. over My Life through:

Revelation	
Understanding	
Love	
Empowerment	

Exercise	
Nutrition	
Journal Notes	
Sealant	

The law of truth was in [Levi's] mouth, and unrighteousness was not found in his lips. Malachi 2:6

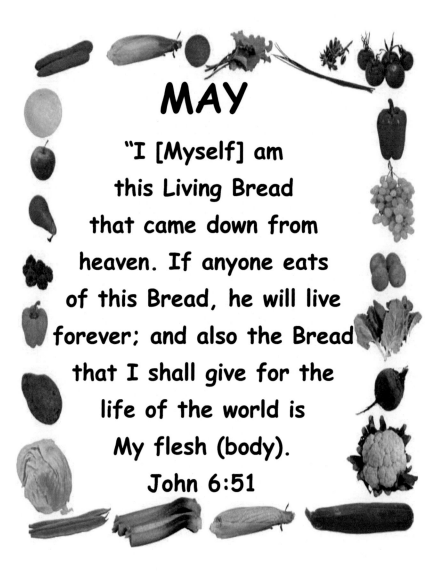

MAY

"I [Myself] am
this Living Bread
that came down from
heaven. If anyone eats
of this Bread, he will live
forever; and also the Bread
that I shall give for the
life of the world is
My flesh (body).
John 6:51

May 1, _____   Day Start _____   End _____

My Prayer Focus _____

_____

Steward of My Spirit Man _____

_____

Steward of My Temple _____

_____

Steward of My Gifts _____

_____

Today I R.U.L.E. over My Life through:

Revelation	
Understanding	
Love	
Empowerment	

Exercise	
Nutrition	
Journal Notes	
Sealant	

Give us this day our daily bread. Matthew 6:11

May 2, _____   Day Start _____   End _____

My Prayer Focus _____

_____

Steward of My Spirit Man _____

_____

Steward of My Temple _____

_____

Steward of My Gifts _____

_____

Today I R.U.L.E. over My Life through:

Revelation	
Understanding	
Love	
Empowerment	

Exercise	
Nutrition	
Journal Notes	
Sealant	

He took bread and, giving thanks to God before them all, he broke it and began to eat. Acts 27:35

May 3, _____   Day Start _____   End _____

My Prayer Focus _____

_____

Steward of My Spirit Man _____

_____

Steward of My Temple _____

_____

Steward of My Gifts _____

_____

Today I R.U.L.E. over My Life through:

Revelation	
Understanding	
Love	
Empowerment	

Exercise	
Nutrition	
Journal Notes	
Sealant	

The bread which we break, does it not mean [that in eating it] we participate in and share a fellowship... 1 Corinthians 10:16

May 4, _____ Day Start _____ End _____

My Prayer Focus _____

_____

Steward of My Spirit Man _____

_____

Steward of My Temple _____

_____

Steward of My Gifts _____

_____

Today I R.U.L.E. over My Life through:

Revelation	
Understanding	
Love	
Empowerment	

Exercise	
Nutrition	
Journal Notes	
Sealant	

May 5, _____ Day Start _____ End _____

My Prayer Focus _____

_____

Steward of My Spirit Man _____

_____

Steward of My Temple _____

_____

Steward of My Gifts _____

_____

Today I R.U.L.E. over My Life through:

Revelation	
Understanding	
Love	
Empowerment	

Exercise	
Nutrition	
Journal Notes	
Sealant	

May 6, _____ Day Start _____ End _____

My Prayer Focus _____

_____

Steward of My Spirit Man _____

_____

Steward of My Temple _____

_____

Steward of My Gifts _____

_____

Today I R.U.L.E. over My Life through:

Revelation	
Understanding	
Love	
Empowerment	

Exercise	
Nutrition	
Journal Notes	
Sealant	

Come, eat of my bread and drink of the [spiritual] wine which I have mixed. Proverbs 9:5

May 7, _____ Day Start _____ End _____

My Prayer Focus _____

_____

Steward of My Spirit Man _____

_____

Steward of My Temple _____

_____

Steward of My Gifts _____

_____

Today I R.U.L.E. over My Life through:

Revelation	
Understanding	
Love	
Empowerment	

Exercise	
Nutrition	
Journal Notes	
Sealant	

May 8, _____   Day Start _____   End _____

My Prayer Focus _____

_____

Steward of My Spirit Man _____

_____

Steward of My Temple _____

_____

Steward of My Gifts _____

_____

Today I R.U.L.E. over My Life through:

Revelation	
Understanding	
Love	
Empowerment	

Exercise	
Nutrition	
Journal Notes	
Sealant	

May 9, _____ Day Start _____ End _____

My Prayer Focus _____

_____

Steward of My Spirit Man _____

_____

Steward of My Temple _____

_____

Steward of My Gifts _____

_____

Today I R.U.L.E. over My Life through:

Revelation	
Understanding	
Love	
Empowerment	

Exercise	
Nutrition	
Journal Notes	
Sealant	

Yet have I not seen the [uncompromisingly] righteous forsaken or their seed begging bread. Psalm 37:25

May 10, _____ Day Start _____ End _____

My Prayer Focus _____

_____

Steward of My Spirit Man _____

_____

Steward of My Temple _____

_____

Steward of My Gifts _____

_____

Today I R.U.L.E. over My Life through:

Revelation	
Understanding	
Love	
Empowerment	

Exercise	
Nutrition	
Journal Notes	
Sealant	

May 11, _____ Day Start _____ End _____

My Prayer Focus _____

_____

Steward of My Spirit Man _____

_____

Steward of My Temple _____

_____

Steward of My Gifts _____

_____

Today I R.U.L.E. over My Life through:

Revelation	
Understanding	
Love	
Empowerment	

Exercise	
Nutrition	
Journal Notes	
Sealant	

May 12, ____ Day Start ____ End ____

My Prayer Focus ______________________________

____

Steward of My Spirit Man ______________________

____

Steward of My Temple _________________________

____

Steward of My Gifts __________________________

____

Today I R.U.L.E. over My Life through:

Revelation	
Understanding	
Love	
Empowerment	

Exercise	
Nutrition	
Journal Notes	
Sealant	

It is not right (proper, becoming, or fair) to take the children's bread and throw it to the little dogs. Matthew 15:26

May 13, _____ Day Start _____ End _____

My Prayer Focus _____

_____

Steward of My Spirit Man _____

_____

Steward of My Temple _____

_____

Steward of My Gifts _____

_____

Today I R.U.L.E. over My Life through:

Revelation	
Understanding	
Love	
Empowerment	

Exercise	
Nutrition	
Journal Notes	
Sealant	

Eat not the bread of him who has a hard, grudging, and envious eye, neither desire his dainty foods. Proverbs 23:6

May 14, _____ Day Start _____ End _____

My Prayer Focus _____

_____

Steward of My Spirit Man _____

_____

Steward of My Temple _____

_____

Steward of My Gifts _____

_____

Today I R.U.L.E. over My Life through:

Revelation	
Understanding	
Love	
Empowerment	

Exercise	
Nutrition	
Journal Notes	
Sealant	

The bread of idleness (gossip discontent, and self-pity) she will not eat. Proverbs 31:27

May 15, _____ Day Start _____ End _____

My Prayer Focus _____

_____

Steward of My Spirit Man _____

_____

Steward of My Temple _____

_____

Steward of My Gifts _____

_____

Today I R.U.L.E. over My Life through:

Revelation	
Understanding	
Love	
Empowerment	

Exercise	
Nutrition	
Journal Notes	
Sealant	

He who tills his land shall be satisfied with bread, but he who follows worthless pursuits is lacking in sense. Proverbs 12:11

May 16, _____ Day Start _____ End _____

My Prayer Focus _____

_____

Steward of My Spirit Man _____

_____

Steward of My Temple _____

_____

Steward of My Gifts _____

_____

Today I R.U.L.E. over My Life through:

Revelation	
Understanding	
Love	
Empowerment	

Exercise	
Nutrition	
Journal Notes	
Sealant	

The Lord gives you the bread of adversity and the water of affliction, yet your Teacher will not hide Himself any more. Isaiah 30:20

May 17, _____ Day Start _____ End _____

My Prayer Focus _____

_____

Steward of My Spirit Man _____

_____

Steward of My Temple _____

_____

Steward of My Gifts _____

_____

Today I R.U.L.E. over My Life through:

Revelation	
Understanding	
Love	
Empowerment	

Exercise	
Nutrition	
Journal Notes	
Sealant	

The words of a talebearer are as wounds, and they go down into the innermost parts of the belly. Proverbs 18:8 KJV

May 18, _____   Day Start _____   End _____

My Prayer Focus _____

_____

Steward of My Spirit Man _____

_____

Steward of My Temple _____

_____

Steward of My Gifts _____

_____

Today I R.U.L.E. over My Life through:

Revelation	
Understanding	
Love	
Empowerment	

Exercise	
Nutrition	
Journal Notes	
Sealant	

May 19, _____ Day Start _____ End _____

My Prayer Focus _____

_____

Steward of My Spirit Man _____

_____

Steward of My Temple _____

_____

Steward of My Gifts _____

_____

Today I R.U.L.E. over My Life through:

Revelation	
Understanding	
Love	
Empowerment	

Exercise	
Nutrition	
Journal Notes	
Sealant	

How is it that you fail to understand that I was not talking to you about bread? Matthew 16:11

May 20, _____ Day Start _____ End _____

My Prayer Focus _____

_____

Steward of My Spirit Man _____

_____

Steward of My Temple _____

_____

Steward of My Gifts _____

_____

Today I R.U.L.E. over My Life through:

Revelation	
Understanding	
Love	
Empowerment	

Exercise	
Nutrition	
Journal Notes	
Sealant	

Now as they were eating, Jesus took bread and, praising God, gave thanks. Matthew 26:26

May 21, _____ Day Start _____ End _____

My Prayer Focus _____

_____

Steward of My Spirit Man _____

_____

Steward of My Temple _____

_____

Steward of My Gifts _____

_____

Today I R.U.L.E. over My Life through:

Revelation	
Understanding	
Love	
Empowerment	

Exercise	
Nutrition	
Journal Notes	
Sealant	

The Lord is my Shepherd [to feed, guide, and shield me], I shall not lack. Psalm 23:1

May 22, _____   Day Start _____   End _____

My Prayer Focus _____

_____

Steward of My Spirit Man _____

_____

Steward of My Temple _____

_____

Steward of My Gifts _____

_____

Today I R.U.L.E. over My Life through:

Revelation	
Understanding	
Love	
Empowerment	

Exercise	
Nutrition	
Journal Notes	
Sealant	

May 23, _____   Day Start _____   End _____

My Prayer Focus _____

_____

Steward of My Spirit Man _____

_____

Steward of My Temple _____

_____

Steward of My Gifts _____

_____

Today I R.U.L.E. over My Life through:

Revelation	
Understanding	
Love	
Empowerment	

Exercise	
Nutrition	
Journal Notes	
Sealant	

May 24, _____ Day Start _____ End _____

My Prayer Focus _____
_____

Steward of My Spirit Man _____
_____

Steward of My Temple _____
_____

Steward of My Gifts _____
_____

Today I R.U.L.E. over My Life through:

Revelation	
Understanding	
Love	
Empowerment	

Exercise	
Nutrition	
Journal Notes	
Sealant	

I also gave you cleanness of teeth in all your cities and want of bread in all your places; yet you did not return to Me. Amos 4:6

May 25, _____ Day Start _____ End _____

My Prayer Focus _____

_____

Steward of My Spirit Man _____

_____

Steward of My Temple _____

_____

Steward of My Gifts _____

_____

Today I R.U.L.E. over My Life through:

Revelation	
Understanding	
Love	
Empowerment	

Exercise	
Nutrition	
Journal Notes	
Sealant	

Nor did we eat anyone's bread without paying for it, but with toil and struggle we worked night and day. 2 Thessalonians 3:8 KJV

May 26, _____ Day Start _____ End _____

My Prayer Focus _____

_____

Steward of My Spirit Man _____

_____

Steward of My Temple _____

_____

Steward of My Gifts _____

_____

Today I R.U.L.E. over My Life through:

Revelation	
Understanding	
Love	
Empowerment	

Exercise	
Nutrition	
Journal Notes	
Sealant	

May 27, _____ Day Start _____ End _____

My Prayer Focus _____

_____

Steward of My Spirit Man _____

_____

Steward of My Temple _____

_____

Steward of My Gifts _____

_____

Today I R.U.L.E. over My Life through:

Revelation	
Understanding	
Love	
Empowerment	

Exercise		
Nutrition		
Journal Notes		
Sealant		

It is vain for you to rise up early, to take rest late, to eat the bread of [anxious] toil...Psalm 127:2

May 28, _____   Day Start _____   End _____

My Prayer Focus _____

_____

Steward of My Spirit Man _____

_____

Steward of My Temple _____

_____

Steward of My Gifts _____

_____

Today I R.U.L.E. over My Life through:

Revelation	
Understanding	
Love	
Empowerment	

Exercise	
Nutrition	
Journal Notes	
Sealant	

May 29, ____ Day Start ____ End ____

My Prayer Focus _____

_____

Steward of My Spirit Man _____

_____

Steward of My Temple _____

_____

Steward of My Gifts _____

_____

Today I R.U.L.E. over My Life through:

Revelation	
Understanding	
Love	
Empowerment	

Exercise	
Nutrition	
Journal Notes	
Sealant	

He distributed to everyone of Israel, both man and woman, to everyone a loaf of bread...1 Chronicles 16:3

May 30, _____   Day Start _____   End _____

My Prayer Focus _____

_____

Steward of My Spirit Man _____

_____

Steward of My Temple _____

_____

Steward of My Gifts _____

_____

Today I R.U.L.E. over My Life through:

Revelation	
Understanding	
Love	
Empowerment	

Exercise	
Nutrition	
Journal Notes	
Sealant	

May 31, _____ Day Start _____ End _____

My Prayer Focus _____

_____

Steward of My Spirit Man _____

_____

Steward of My Temple _____

_____

Steward of My Gifts _____

_____

Today I R.U.L.E. over My Life through:

Revelation	
Understanding	
Love	
Empowerment	

Exercise	
Nutrition	
Journal Notes	
Sealant	

He brought quails and satisfied them with the bread of heaven. Psalm 105:40

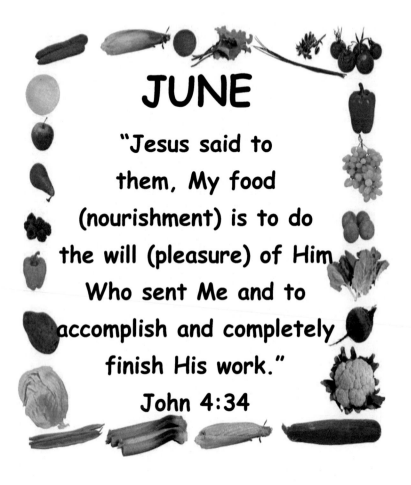

JUNE

"Jesus said to them, My food (nourishment) is to do the will (pleasure) of Him Who sent Me and to accomplish and completely finish His work."

John 4:34

June 1, _____ Day Start ____ End ____

My Prayer Focus _____

_____

Steward of My Spirit Man _____

_____

Steward of My Temple _____

_____

Steward of My Gifts _____

_____

Today I R.U.L.E. over My Life through:

Revelation	
Understanding	
Love	
Empowerment	

Exercise	
Nutrition	
Journal Notes	
Sealant	

Let your light so shine before men, that they may see your good works, and glorify your Father...in heaven. Matthew 5:16 KJV

June 2, _____ Day Start _____ End _____

My Prayer Focus _____

_____

Steward of My Spirit Man _____

_____

Steward of My Temple _____

_____

Steward of My Gifts _____

_____

Today I R.U.L.E. over My Life through:

Revelation	
Understanding	
Love	
Empowerment	

Exercise	
Nutrition	
Journal Notes	
Sealant	

For we are his workmanship, created in Christ Jesus unto good works... Ephesians 2:10

June 3, _____ Day Start ____ End ____

My Prayer Focus _____

_____

Steward of My Spirit Man _____

_____

Steward of My Temple _____

_____

Steward of My Gifts _____

_____

Today I R.U.L.E. over My Life through:

Revelation	
Understanding	
Love	
Empowerment	

Exercise	
Nutrition	
Journal Notes	
Sealant	

...which God hath before ordained that we should walk in them. Ephesians 2:10

June 4, _____ Day Start _____ End _____

My Prayer Focus _____

_____

Steward of My Spirit Man _____

_____

Steward of My Temple _____

_____

Steward of My Gifts _____

_____

Today I R.U.L.E. over My Life through:

Revelation	
Understanding	
Love	
Empowerment	

Exercise	
Nutrition	
Journal Notes	
Sealant	

June 5, _____ Day Start _____ End _____

My Prayer Focus _____

_____

Steward of My Spirit Man _____

_____

Steward of My Temple _____

_____

Steward of My Gifts _____

_____

Today I R.U.L.E. over My Life through:

Revelation	
Understanding	
Love	
Empowerment	

Exercise	
Nutrition	
Journal Notes	
Sealant	

We must work the works of Him Who sent Me and be busy with His business while it is daylight...John 9:4

June 6, _____ Day Start _____ End _____

My Prayer Focus _____

_____

Steward of My Spirit Man _____

_____

Steward of My Temple _____

_____

Steward of My Gifts _____

_____

Today I R.U.L.E. over My Life through:

Revelation	
Understanding	
Love	
Empowerment	

Exercise	
Nutrition	
Journal Notes	
Sealant	

June 7, _____ Day Start _____ End _____

My Prayer Focus _____

_____

Steward of My Spirit Man _____

_____

Steward of My Temple _____

_____

Steward of My Gifts _____

_____

Today I R.U.L.E. over My Life through:

Revelation	
Understanding	
Love	
Empowerment	

Exercise	
Nutrition	
Journal Notes	
Sealant	

And he will shew him greater works than these, that ye may marvel. John 5:20 KJV

June 8, _____ Day Start _____ End _____

My Prayer Focus _____

_____

Steward of My Spirit Man _____

_____

Steward of My Temple _____

_____

Steward of My Gifts _____

_____

Today I R.U.L.E. over My Life through:

Revelation	
Understanding	
Love	
Empowerment	

Exercise	
Nutrition	
Journal Notes	
Sealant	

June 9, _____ Day Start _____ End _____

My Prayer Focus _____

_____

Steward of My Spirit Man _____

_____

Steward of My Temple _____

_____

Steward of My Gifts _____

_____

Today I R.U.L.E. over My Life through:

Revelation	
Understanding	
Love	
Empowerment	

Exercise	
Nutrition	
Journal Notes	
Sealant	

Lord, You will ordain peace...for us, for You have also wrought in us and for us all our works. Isaiah 26:12

June 10, _____ Day Start ____ End ____

My Prayer Focus _____

_____

Steward of My Spirit Man _____

_____

Steward of My Temple _____

_____

Steward of My Gifts _____

_____

Today I R.U.L.E. over My Life through:

Revelation	
Understanding	
Love	
Empowerment	

Exercise	
Nutrition	
Journal Notes	
Sealant	

Your mercy and loving-kindness, O Lord, endure forever--forsake not the works of Your own hands. Psalm 138:8

June 11, _____ Day Start _____ End _____

My Prayer Focus _____

_____

Steward of My Spirit Man _____

_____

Steward of My Temple _____

_____

Steward of My Gifts _____

_____

Today I R.U.L.E. over My Life through:

Revelation	
Understanding	
Love	
Empowerment	

Exercise	
Nutrition	
Journal Notes	
Sealant	

Wonderful are Your works, and that my inner self knows right well. Psalm 139:14

June 12, _____ Day Start _____ End _____

My Prayer Focus _____

_____

Steward of My Spirit Man _____

_____

Steward of My Temple _____

_____

Steward of My Gifts _____

_____

Today I R.U.L.E. over My Life through:

Revelation	
Understanding	
Love	
Empowerment	

Exercise	
Nutrition	
Journal Notes	
Sealant	

For the Lord your God has blessed you in all the work of your hand. Deuteronomy 2:7

June 13, _____ Day Start _____ End _____

My Prayer Focus _____

_____

Steward of My Spirit Man _____

_____

Steward of My Temple _____

_____

Steward of My Gifts _____

_____

Today I R.U.L.E. over My Life through:

Revelation	
Understanding	
Love	
Empowerment	

Exercise	
Nutrition	
Journal Notes	
Sealant	

June 14, _____ Day Start _____ End _____

My Prayer Focus _____

_____

Steward of My Spirit Man _____

_____

Steward of My Temple _____

_____

Steward of My Gifts _____

_____

Today I R.U.L.E. over My Life through:

Revelation	
Understanding	
Love	
Empowerment	

Exercise	
Nutrition	
Journal Notes	
Sealant	

For God is not unrighteous to forget your work and labour of love, which ye have shewed toward his name... Hebrews 6:10 KJV

June 15, _____ Day Start _____ End _____

My Prayer Focus _____

_____

Steward of My Spirit Man _____

_____

Steward of My Temple _____

_____

Steward of My Gifts _____

_____

Today I R.U.L.E. over My Life through:

Revelation	
Understanding	
Love	
Empowerment	

Exercise		
Nutrition		
Journal Notes		
Sealant		

June 16, _____ Day Start _____ End _____

My Prayer Focus _____

_____

Steward of My Spirit Man _____

_____

Steward of My Temple _____

_____

Steward of My Gifts _____

_____

Today I R.U.L.E. over My Life through:

Revelation	
Understanding	
Love	
Empowerment	

Exercise	
Nutrition	
Journal Notes	
Sealant	

June 17, _____ Day Start _____ End _____

My Prayer Focus _____

_____

Steward of My Spirit Man _____

_____

Steward of My Temple _____

_____

Steward of My Gifts _____

_____

Today I R.U.L.E. over My Life through:

Revelation	
Understanding	
Love	
Empowerment	

Exercise	
Nutrition	
Journal Notes	
Sealant	

He Who began a good work in you will continue until the day of Jesus Christ...Philippians 1:6

June 18, _____ Day Start _____ End _____

My Prayer Focus _____

_____

Steward of My Spirit Man _____

_____

Steward of My Temple _____

_____

Steward of My Gifts _____

_____

Today I R.U.L.E. over My Life through:

Revelation	
Understanding	
Love	
Empowerment	

Exercise	
Nutrition	
Journal Notes	
Sealant	

...developing [that good work] and perfecting and bringing it to full completion in you. Philippians 1:6

June 19, _____ Day Start _____ End _____

My Prayer Focus _____

_____

Steward of My Spirit Man _____

_____

Steward of My Temple _____

_____

Steward of My Gifts _____

_____

Today I R.U.L.E. over My Life through:

Revelation	
Understanding	
Love	
Empowerment	

Exercise	
Nutrition	
Journal Notes	
Sealant	

June 20, _____ Day Start _____ End _____

My Prayer Focus _____

_____

Steward of My Spirit Man _____

_____

Steward of My Temple _____

_____

Steward of My Gifts _____

_____

Today I R.U.L.E. over My Life through:

Revelation	
Understanding	
Love	
Empowerment	

Exercise	
Nutrition	
Journal Notes	
Sealant	

He being not a forgetful hearer, but a doer of the work, this man shall be blessed in his deed. James 1:25

June 21, _____ Day Start _____ End _____

My Prayer Focus _____

_____

Steward of My Spirit Man _____

_____

Steward of My Temple _____

_____

Steward of My Gifts _____

_____

Today I R.U.L.E. over My Life through:

Revelation	
Understanding	
Love	
Empowerment	

Exercise	
Nutrition	
Journal Notes	
Sealant	

He was not able to do even one work of power there, except that He laid His... sickly people [and] cured them. Mark 6:5

June 22, _____ Day Start _____ End _____

My Prayer Focus _____

_____

Steward of My Spirit Man _____

_____

Steward of My Temple _____

_____

Steward of My Gifts _____

_____

Today I R.U.L.E. over My Life through:

Revelation	
Understanding	
Love	
Empowerment	

Exercise	
Nutrition	
Journal Notes	
Sealant	

For thou, LORD, hast made me glad through thy work: I will triumph in the works of thy hands. Psalm 92:4 KJV

June 23, _____ Day Start _____ End _____

My Prayer Focus _____

_____

Steward of My Spirit Man _____

_____

Steward of My Temple _____

_____

Steward of My Gifts _____

_____

Today I R.U.L.E. over My Life through:

Revelation	
Understanding	
Love	
Empowerment	

Exercise	
Nutrition	
Journal Notes	
Sealant	

That ye, always having all sufficiency in all things, may abound to every good work: 2 Corinthians 9:8 KJV

June 24, _____ Day Start ____ End ____

My Prayer Focus _____

_____

Steward of My Spirit Man _____

_____

Steward of My Temple _____

_____

Steward of My Gifts _____

_____

Today I R.U.L.E. over My Life through:

Revelation	
Understanding	
Love	
Empowerment	

Exercise	
Nutrition	
Journal Notes	
Sealant	

Give her of the fruit of her hands, and let her own works praise her in the gates [of the city]! Proverbs 31:31

June 25, _____ Day Start _____ End _____

My Prayer Focus _____

_____

Steward of My Spirit Man _____

_____

Steward of My Temple _____

_____

Steward of My Gifts _____

_____

Today I R.U.L.E. over My Life through:

Revelation	
Understanding	
Love	
Empowerment	

Exercise	
Nutrition	
Journal Notes	
Sealant	

June 26, _____ Day Start _____ End _____

My Prayer Focus _____

_____

Steward of My Spirit Man _____

_____

Steward of My Temple _____

_____

Steward of My Gifts _____

_____

Today I R.U.L.E. over My Life through:

Revelation	
Understanding	
Love	
Empowerment	

Exercise	
Nutrition	
Journal Notes	
Sealant	

Consider the work of God: who can make straight what He has made crooked? Ecclesiastes 7:13

June 27, _____ Day Start _____ End _____

My Prayer Focus _____

_____

Steward of My Spirit Man _____

_____

Steward of My Temple _____

_____

Steward of My Gifts _____

_____

Today I R.U.L.E. over My Life through:

Revelation	
Understanding	
Love	
Empowerment	

Exercise	
Nutrition	
Journal Notes	
Sealant	

June 28, _____ Day Start _____ End _____

My Prayer Focus _____

_____

Steward of My Spirit Man _____

_____

Steward of My Temple _____

_____

Steward of My Gifts _____

_____

Today I R.U.L.E. over My Life through:

Revelation	
Understanding	
Love	
Empowerment	

Exercise	
Nutrition	
Journal Notes	
Sealant	

But let every person carefully scrutinize and examine and test his own conduct and his own work. Galatians 6:4

June 29, _____ Day Start _____ End _____

My Prayer Focus _____

_____

Steward of My Spirit Man _____

_____

Steward of My Temple _____

_____

Steward of My Gifts _____

_____

Today I R.U.L.E. over My Life through:

Revelation	
Understanding	
Love	
Empowerment	

Exercise	
Nutrition	
Journal Notes	
Sealant	

God blessed (spoke good of) the seventh day, set it apart as His own.... God rested from all His work. Genesis 2:3

June 30, _____ Day Start _____ End _____

My Prayer Focus _____

_____

Steward of My Spirit Man _____

_____

Steward of My Temple _____

_____

Steward of My Gifts _____

_____

Today I R.U.L.E. over My Life through:

Revelation	
Understanding	
Love	
Empowerment	

Exercise	
Nutrition	
Journal Notes	
Sealant	

LOVE

RULE No. 3

LOVE
MUST BE MY DECIDING
FACTOR

*He said to him the third time,
Simon, son of John, do you love
Me [with a deep, instinctive, personal
affection for Me, as for a close friend]?
Peter was grieved (was saddened and hurt)
that He should ask him the third time, Do you
love Me? And he said to Him, Lord, You know
everything; You know that I love You [that I
have a deep, instinctive, personal affection
for You, as for a close friend]. Jesus
said to him, Feed My sheep.
John 21:17*

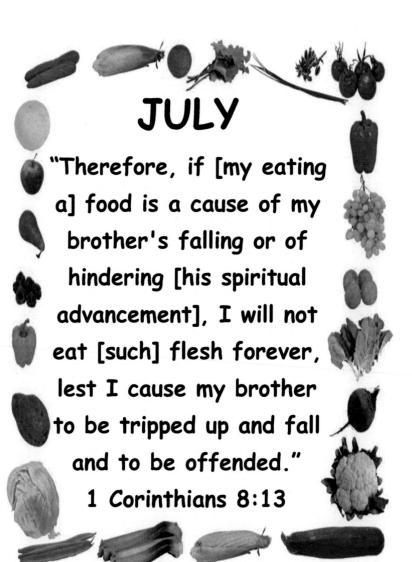

JULY

"Therefore, if [my eating a] food is a cause of my brother's falling or of hindering [his spiritual advancement], I will not eat [such] flesh forever, lest I cause my brother to be tripped up and fall and to be offended."

1 Corinthians 8:13

July 1, _____ Day Start _____ End _____

My Prayer Focus _____

_____

Steward of My Spirit Man _____

_____

Steward of My Temple _____

_____

Steward of My Gifts _____

_____

Today I R.U.L.E. over My Life through:

Revelation	
Understanding	
Love	
Empowerment	

Exercise	
Nutrition	
Journal Notes	
Sealant	

July 2, _____ Day Start _____ End _____

My Prayer Focus _____

_____

Steward of My Spirit Man _____

_____

Steward of My Temple _____

_____

Steward of My Gifts _____

_____

Today I R.U.L.E. over My Life through:

Revelation	
Understanding	
Love	
Empowerment	

Exercise	
Nutrition	
Journal Notes	
Sealant	

But I tell you, Love your enemies and pray for those who persecute you. Matthew 5:44

July 3, _____ Day Start _____ End _____

My Prayer Focus _____

_____

Steward of My Spirit Man _____

_____

Steward of My Temple _____

_____

Steward of My Gifts _____

_____

Today I R.U.L.E. over My Life through:

Revelation	
Understanding	
Love	
Empowerment	

Exercise	
Nutrition	
Journal Notes	
Sealant	

July 4, _____ Day Start _____ End _____

My Prayer Focus _____

_____

Steward of My Spirit Man _____

_____

Steward of My Temple _____

_____

Steward of My Gifts _____

_____

Today I R.U.L.E. over My Life through:

Revelation	
Understanding	
Love	
Empowerment	

Exercise	
Nutrition	
Journal Notes	
Sealant	

Let love for your fellow believers continue and be a fixed practice with you [never let it fail]. Hebrews 13:1

July 5, _____ Day Start _____ End _____

My Prayer Focus _____

_____

Steward of My Spirit Man _____

_____

Steward of My Temple _____

_____

Steward of My Gifts _____

_____

Today I R.U.L.E. over My Life through:

Revelation	
Understanding	
Love	
Empowerment	

Exercise	
Nutrition	
Journal Notes	
Sealant	

[Let your] love be sincere (a real thing); hate what is evil [loathe all ungodliness, turn in horror from wickedness]. Romans 12:9

July 6, _____ Day Start _____ End _____

My Prayer Focus _____

_____

Steward of My Spirit Man _____

_____

Steward of My Temple _____

_____

Steward of My Gifts _____

_____

Today I R.U.L.E. over My Life through:

Revelation	
Understanding	
Love	
Empowerment	

Exercise	
Nutrition	
Journal Notes	
Sealant	

July 7, _____ Day Start _____ End _____

My Prayer Focus _____

_____

Steward of My Spirit Man _____

_____

Steward of My Temple _____

_____

Steward of My Gifts _____

_____

Today I R.U.L.E. over My Life through:

Revelation	
Understanding	
Love	
Empowerment	

Exercise	
Nutrition	
Journal Notes	
Sealant	

Complete my joy by living in harmony and being of the same mind and one in purpose, having the same love. Philippians 2:2

July 8, _____ Day Start _____ End _____

My Prayer Focus _____

_____

Steward of My Spirit Man _____

_____

Steward of My Temple _____

_____

Steward of My Gifts _____

_____

Today I R.U.L.E. over My Life through:

Revelation	
Understanding	
Love	
Empowerment	

Exercise	
Nutrition	
Journal Notes	
Sealant	

For this is the message (the announcement) which you have heard from the first, that we should love one another. 1 John 3:11

July 9, _____ Day Start _____ End _____

My Prayer Focus _____

_____

Steward of My Spirit Man _____

_____

Steward of My Temple _____

_____

Steward of My Gifts _____

_____

Today I R.U.L.E. over My Life through:

Revelation	
Understanding	
Love	
Empowerment	

Exercise	
Nutrition	
Journal Notes	
Sealant	

July 10, _____ Day Start _____ End _____

My Prayer Focus _____

_____

Steward of My Spirit Man _____

_____

Steward of My Temple _____

_____

Steward of My Gifts _____

_____

Today I R.U.L.E. over My Life through:

Revelation	
Understanding	
Love	
Empowerment	

Exercise	
Nutrition	
Journal Notes	
Sealant	

Faith activated and energized and expressed and working through love. Galatians 5:6

July 11, _____ Day Start _____ End _____

My Prayer Focus _____

_____

Steward of My Spirit Man _____

_____

Steward of My Temple _____

_____

Steward of My Gifts _____

_____

Today I R.U.L.E. over My Life through:

Revelation	
Understanding	
Love	
Empowerment	

Exercise	
Nutrition	
Journal Notes	
Sealant	

July 12, _____ Day Start _____ End _____

My Prayer Focus _____

_____

Steward of My Spirit Man _____

_____

Steward of My Temple _____

_____

Steward of My Gifts _____

_____

Today I R.U.L.E. over My Life through:

Revelation	
Understanding	
Love	
Empowerment	

Exercise	
Nutrition	
Journal Notes	
Sealant	

I have loved you with an everlasting love; therefore with loving-kindness have I drawn you. Jeremiah 31:3

July 13, _____ Day Start ____ End ____

My Prayer Focus _____

_____

Steward of My Spirit Man _____

_____

Steward of My Temple _____

_____

Steward of My Gifts _____

_____

Today I R.U.L.E. over My Life through:

Revelation	
Understanding	
Love	
Empowerment	

Exercise	
Nutrition	
Journal Notes	
Sealant	

But God commendeth his love toward us, in that, while we were yet sinners, Christ died for us. Romans 5:8 KJV

July 14, _____ Day Start _____ End _____

My Prayer Focus _____

_____

Steward of My Spirit Man _____

_____

Steward of My Temple _____

_____

Steward of My Gifts _____

_____

Today I R.U.L.E. over My Life through:

Revelation	
Understanding	
Love	
Empowerment	

Exercise	
Nutrition	
Journal Notes	
Sealant	

No one has greater love [no one has shown stronger affection] than to lay down (give up) his own life for his friends. John 5:13

July 15, _____ Day Start _____ End _____

My Prayer Focus _____

_____

Steward of My Spirit Man _____

_____

Steward of My Temple _____

_____

Steward of My Gifts _____

_____

Today I R.U.L.E. over My Life through:

Revelation	
Understanding	
Love	
Empowerment	

Exercise	
Nutrition	
Journal Notes	
Sealant	

With patience, bearing with one another and making allowances because you love one another. Ephesians 4:2

July 16, _____ Day Start _____ End _____

My Prayer Focus _____

_____

Steward of My Spirit Man _____

_____

Steward of My Temple _____

_____

Steward of My Gifts _____

_____

Today I R.U.L.E. over My Life through:

Revelation	
Understanding	
Love	
Empowerment	

Exercise	
Nutrition	
Journal Notes	
Sealant	

Let our lives lovingly express truth [in all things, speaking truly, dealing truly, living truly]. Enfolded in love... Ephesians 4:15

July 17, _____ Day Start _____ End _____

My Prayer Focus _____

_____

Steward of My Spirit Man _____

_____

Steward of My Temple _____

_____

Steward of My Gifts _____

_____

Today I R.U.L.E. over My Life through:

Revelation	
Understanding	
Love	
Empowerment	

Exercise	
Nutrition	
Journal Notes	
Sealant	

For the love of Christ compels us, because we judge thus: that if One died for all, then all died. 2 Corinthians 5:14 NKJV

July 18, _____ Day Start _____ End _____

My Prayer Focus _____

_____

Steward of My Spirit Man _____

_____

Steward of My Temple _____

_____

Steward of My Gifts _____

_____

Today I R.U.L.E. over My Life through:

Revelation	
Understanding	
Love	
Empowerment	

Exercise	
Nutrition	
Journal Notes	
Sealant	

July 19, _____ Day Start ____ End ____

My Prayer Focus _____

_____

Steward of My Spirit Man _____

_____

Steward of My Temple _____

_____

Steward of My Gifts _____

_____

Today I R.U.L.E. over My Life through:

Revelation	
Understanding	
Love	
Empowerment	

Exercise	
Nutrition	
Journal Notes	
Sealant	

July 20, _____ Day Start _____ End _____

My Prayer Focus _____

_____

Steward of My Spirit Man _____

_____

Steward of My Temple _____

_____

Steward of My Gifts _____

_____

Today I R.U.L.E. over My Life through:

Revelation	
Understanding	
Love	
Empowerment	

Exercise	
Nutrition	
Journal Notes	
Sealant	

May the Lord make you to increase and excel and overflow in love for one another and for all people. 1 Thessalonians 3:12

July 21, _____ Day Start _____ End _____

My Prayer Focus _____

_____

Steward of My Spirit Man _____

_____

Steward of My Temple _____

_____

Steward of My Gifts _____

_____

Today I R.U.L.E. over My Life through:

Revelation	
Understanding	
Love	
Empowerment	

Exercise	
Nutrition	
Journal Notes	
Sealant	

He who does not love has not become acquainted with God [does not and never did know Him], for God is love. 1 John 4:8

July 22, _____ Day Start _____ End _____

My Prayer Focus _____

_____

Steward of My Spirit Man _____

_____

Steward of My Temple _____

_____

Steward of My Gifts _____

_____

Today I R.U.L.E. over My Life through:

Revelation	
Understanding	
Love	
Empowerment	

Exercise	
Nutrition	
Journal Notes	
Sealant	

July 23, _____ Day Start _____ End _____

My Prayer Focus _____

_____

Steward of My Spirit Man _____

_____

Steward of My Temple _____

_____

Steward of My Gifts _____

_____

Today I R.U.L.E. over My Life through:

Revelation	
Understanding	
Love	
Empowerment	

Exercise	
Nutrition	
Journal Notes	
Sealant	

July 24, _____ Day Start _____ End _____

My Prayer Focus _____

_____

Steward of My Spirit Man _____

_____

Steward of My Temple _____

_____

Steward of My Gifts _____

_____

Today I R.U.L.E. over My Life through:

Revelation	
Understanding	
Love	
Empowerment	

Exercise	
Nutrition	
Journal Notes	
Sealant	

July 25, _____ Day Start _____ End _____

My Prayer Focus _____

_____

Steward of My Spirit Man _____

_____

Steward of My Temple _____

_____

Steward of My Gifts _____

_____

Today I R.U.L.E. over My Life through:

Revelation	
Understanding	
Love	
Empowerment	

Exercise	
Nutrition	
Journal Notes	
Sealant	

You love righteousness, uprightness, and right standing with God and hate wickedness... Your God, has anointed you. Psalm 45:7

July 26, _____ Day Start _____ End _____

My Prayer Focus _____

_____

Steward of My Spirit Man _____

_____

Steward of My Temple _____

_____

Steward of My Gifts _____

_____

Today I R.U.L.E. over My Life through:

Revelation	
Understanding	
Love	
Empowerment	

Exercise	
Nutrition	
Journal Notes	
Sealant	

Hearing of thy love and faith, which thou hast toward the Lord Jesus, and toward all saints. Philemon 4 KJV

July 27, _____ Day Start _____ End _____

My Prayer Focus _____

_____

Steward of My Spirit Man _____

_____

Steward of My Temple _____

_____

Steward of My Gifts _____

_____

Today I R.U.L.E. over My Life through:

Revelation	
Understanding	
Love	
Empowerment	

Exercise	
Nutrition	
Journal Notes	
Sealant	

There is no fear in love; but perfect love casteth out fear: because fear hath torment. 1 John 4:18

July 28, _____ Day Start _____ End _____

My Prayer Focus _____

_____

Steward of My Spirit Man _____

_____

Steward of My Temple _____

_____

Steward of My Gifts _____

_____

Today I R.U.L.E. over My Life through:

Revelation	
Understanding	
Love	
Empowerment	

Exercise	
Nutrition	
Journal Notes	
Sealant	

For if you love those who love you, what reward can you have? Matthew 5:46

July 29, _____ Day Start _____ End _____

My Prayer Focus _____

_____

Steward of My Spirit Man _____

_____

Steward of My Temple _____

_____

Steward of My Gifts _____

_____

Today I R.U.L.E. over My Life through:

Revelation	
Understanding	
Love	
Empowerment	

Exercise	
Nutrition	
Journal Notes	
Sealant	

Love not sleep, lest you come to poverty; open your eyes and you will be satisfied with bread. Proverbs 20:13

July 30, _____ Day Start _____ End _____

My Prayer Focus _____

_____

Steward of My Spirit Man _____

_____

Steward of My Temple _____

_____

Steward of My Gifts _____

_____

Today I R.U.L.E. over My Life through:

Revelation	
Understanding	
Love	
Empowerment	

Exercise	
Nutrition	
Journal Notes	
Sealant	

July 31, _____ Day Start _____ End _____

My Prayer Focus _____

_____

Steward of My Spirit Man _____

_____

Steward of My Temple _____

_____

Steward of My Gifts _____

_____

Today I R.U.L.E. over My Life through:

Revelation	
Understanding	
Love	
Empowerment	

Exercise	
Nutrition	
Journal Notes	
Sealant	

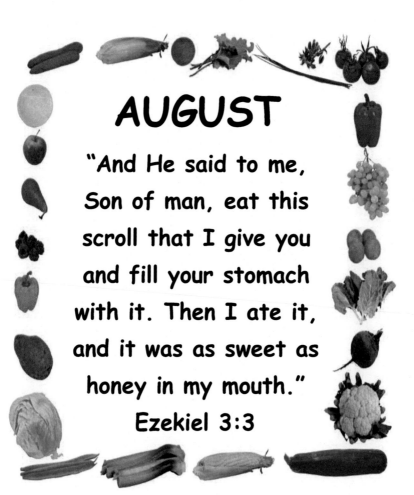

AUGUST

"And He said to me,
Son of man, eat this
scroll that I give you
and fill your stomach
with it. Then I ate it,
and it was as sweet as
honey in my mouth."
Ezekiel 3:3

August 1, _____ Day Start _____ End _____

My Prayer Focus _____

_____

Steward of My Spirit Man _____

_____

Steward of My Temple _____

_____

Steward of My Gifts _____

_____

Today I R.U.L.E. over My Life through:

Revelation	
Understanding	
Love	
Empowerment	

Exercise	
Nutrition	
Journal Notes	
Sealant	

How sweet are Your words to my taste, sweeter than honey to my mouth! Psalm 119:103

August 2, _____ Day Start _____ End _____

My Prayer Focus _____

_____

Steward of My Spirit Man _____

_____

Steward of My Temple _____

_____

Steward of My Gifts _____

_____

Today I R.U.L.E. over My Life through:

Revelation	
Understanding	
Love	
Empowerment	

Exercise	
Nutrition	
Journal Notes	
Sealant	

O taste and see that the Lord [our God] is good! Psalm 34:8

August 3, _____ Day Start _____ End _____

My Prayer Focus _____

_____

Steward of My Spirit Man _____

_____

Steward of My Temple _____

_____

Steward of My Gifts _____

_____

Today I R.U.L.E. over My Life through:

Revelation	
Understanding	
Love	
Empowerment	

Exercise	
Nutrition	
Journal Notes	
Sealant	

My son, eat honey, because it is good, and the drippings of the honeycomb are sweet to your taste. Proverbs 24:13

August 4, _____ Day Start _____ End _____

My Prayer Focus _____

_____

Steward of My Spirit Man _____

_____

Steward of My Temple _____

_____

Steward of My Gifts _____

_____

Today I R.U.L.E. over My Life through:

Revelation	
Understanding	
Love	
Empowerment	

Exercise	
Nutrition	
Journal Notes	
Sealant	

August 5, _____ Day Start _____ End _____

My Prayer Focus _____

_____

Steward of My Spirit Man _____

_____

Steward of My Temple _____

_____

Steward of My Gifts _____

_____

Today I R.U.L.E. over My Life through:

Revelation	
Understanding	
Love	
Empowerment	

Exercise	
Nutrition	
Journal Notes	
Sealant	

August 6, _____ Day Start _____ End _____

My Prayer Focus _____

_____

Steward of My Spirit Man _____

_____

Steward of My Temple _____

_____

Steward of My Gifts _____

_____

Today I R.U.L.E. over My Life through:

Revelation	
Understanding	
Love	
Empowerment	

Exercise	
Nutrition	
Journal Notes	
Sealant	

Take it and eat it. It will embitter your stomach, though in your mouth it will be as sweet as honey. Revelation 10:9

August 7, _____ Day Start _____ End _____

My Prayer Focus _____

_____

Steward of My Spirit Man _____

_____

Steward of My Temple _____

_____

Steward of My Gifts _____

_____

Today I R.U.L.E. over My Life through:

Revelation	
Understanding	
Love	
Empowerment	

Exercise	
Nutrition	
Journal Notes	
Sealant	

It was as sweet as honey in my mouth, but once I had swallowed it, my stomach was embittered. Revelation 10:10

August 8, _____ Day Start _____ End _____

My Prayer Focus _____

_____

Steward of My Spirit Man _____

_____

Steward of My Temple _____

_____

Steward of My Gifts _____

_____

Today I R.U.L.E. over My Life through:

Revelation	
Understanding	
Love	
Empowerment	

Exercise	
Nutrition	
Journal Notes	
Sealant	

August 9, _____ Day Start _____ End _____

My Prayer Focus _____

_____

Steward of My Spirit Man _____

_____

Steward of My Temple _____

_____

Steward of My Gifts _____

_____

Today I R.U.L.E. over My Life through:

Revelation	
Understanding	
Love	
Empowerment	

Exercise	
Nutrition	
Journal Notes	
Sealant	

August 10, _____ Day Start _____ End _____

My Prayer Focus _____

_____

Steward of My Spirit Man _____

_____

Steward of My Temple _____

_____

Steward of My Gifts _____

_____

Today I R.U.L.E. over My Life through:

Revelation	
Understanding	
Love	
Empowerment	

Exercise	
Nutrition	
Journal Notes	
Sealant	

August 11, _____ Day Start _____ End _____

My Prayer Focus _____

_____

Steward of My Spirit Man _____

_____

Steward of My Temple _____

_____

Steward of My Gifts _____

_____

Today I R.U.L.E. over My Life through:

Revelation	
Understanding	
Love	
Empowerment	

Exercise	
Nutrition	
Journal Notes	
Sealant	

August 12, _____ Day Start _____ End _____

My Prayer Focus _____

_____

Steward of My Spirit Man _____

_____

Steward of My Temple _____

_____

Steward of My Gifts _____

_____

Today I R.U.L.E. over My Life through:

Revelation	
Understanding	
Love	
Empowerment	

Exercise	
Nutrition	
Journal Notes	
Sealant	

August 13, _____ Day Start _____ End _____

My Prayer Focus _____

_____

Steward of My Spirit Man _____

_____

Steward of My Temple _____

_____

Steward of My Gifts _____

_____

Today I R.U.L.E. over My Life through:

Revelation	
Understanding	
Love	
Empowerment	

Exercise	
Nutrition	
Journal Notes	
Sealant	

It is not good to eat much honey; so for men to seek glory, their own glory, causes suffering and is not glory. Proverbs 25:27

August 14, _____ Day Start _____ End _____

My Prayer Focus _____

_____

Steward of My Spirit Man _____

_____

Steward of My Temple _____

_____

Steward of My Gifts _____

_____

Today I R.U.L.E. over My Life through:

Revelation	
Understanding	
Love	
Empowerment	

Exercise	
Nutrition	
Journal Notes	
Sealant	

August 15, _____ Day Start _____ End _____

My Prayer Focus _____

_____

Steward of My Spirit Man _____

_____

Steward of My Temple _____

_____

Steward of My Gifts _____

_____

Today I R.U.L.E. over My Life through:

Revelation	
Understanding	
Love	
Empowerment	

Exercise	
Nutrition	
Journal Notes	
Sealant	

As soon as the command went abroad, the Israelites gave in abundance the firstfruits of...honey...2 Chronicles 31:5

August 16, _____ Day Start _____ End _____

My Prayer Focus _____

_____

Steward of My Spirit Man _____

_____

Steward of My Temple _____

_____

Steward of My Gifts _____

_____

Today I R.U.L.E. over My Life through:

Revelation	
Understanding	
Love	
Empowerment	

Exercise	
Nutrition	
Journal Notes	
Sealant	

And of all the produce of the field; and they brought in abundantly the tithe of everything. 2 Chronicles 31:5

August 17, _____ Day Start _____ End _____

My Prayer Focus _____

_____

Steward of My Spirit Man _____

_____

Steward of My Temple _____

_____

Steward of My Gifts _____

_____

Today I R.U.L.E. over My Life through:

Revelation	
Understanding	
Love	
Empowerment	

Exercise	
Nutrition	
Journal Notes	
Sealant	

August 18, _____ Day Start _____ End _____

My Prayer Focus _____

_____

Steward of My Spirit Man _____

_____

Steward of My Temple _____

_____

Steward of My Gifts _____

_____

Today I R.U.L.E. over My Life through:

Revelation	
Understanding	
Love	
Empowerment	

Exercise	
Nutrition	
Journal Notes	
Sealant	

August 19, _____ Day Start _____ End _____

My Prayer Focus _____

_____

Steward of My Spirit Man _____

_____

Steward of My Temple _____

_____

Steward of My Gifts _____

_____

Today I R.U.L.E. over My Life through:

Revelation	
Understanding	
Love	
Empowerment	

Exercise	
Nutrition	
Journal Notes	
Sealant	

For *it is* impossible for those who were once enlightened, and have tasted the heavenly gift...Hebrews 6:4

August 20, _____ Day Start _____ End _____

My Prayer Focus _____

_____

Steward of My Spirit Man _____

_____

Steward of My Temple _____

_____

Steward of My Gifts _____

_____

Today I R.U.L.E. over My Life through:

Revelation	
Understanding	
Love	
Empowerment	

Exercise	
Nutrition	
Journal Notes	
Sealant	

Have become partakers of the Holy Spirit...have tasted the good word of God and the powers of the age to come...Hebrew 6:5

August 21, _____ Day Start _____ End _____

My Prayer Focus _____

_____

Steward of My Spirit Man _____

_____

Steward of My Temple _____

_____

Steward of My Gifts _____

_____

Today I R.U.L.E. over My Life through:

Revelation	
Understanding	
Love	
Empowerment	

Exercise	
Nutrition	
Journal Notes	
Sealant	

If they fall away, to renew them again to repentance, since they crucify again for themselves the Son of God...Hebrews 6:6

August 22, _____ Day Start _____ End _____

My Prayer Focus _____

_____

Steward of My Spirit Man _____

_____

Steward of My Temple _____

_____

Steward of My Gifts _____

_____

Today I R.U.L.E. over My Life through:

Revelation	
Understanding	
Love	
Empowerment	

Exercise	
Nutrition	
Journal Notes	
Sealant	

August 23, _____ Day Start _____ End _____

My Prayer Focus _____

_____

Steward of My Spirit Man _____

_____

Steward of My Temple _____

_____

Steward of My Gifts _____

_____

Today I R.U.L.E. over My Life through:

Revelation	
Understanding	
Love	
Empowerment	

Exercise	
Nutrition	
Journal Notes	
Sealant	

August 24, _____ Day Start _____ End _____

My Prayer Focus _____

_____

Steward of My Spirit Man _____

_____

Steward of My Temple _____

_____

Steward of My Gifts _____

_____

Today I R.U.L.E. over My Life through:

Revelation	
Understanding	
Love	
Empowerment	

Exercise	
Nutrition	
Journal Notes	
Sealant	

Not that which goeth into the mouth defileth a man...which cometh out of the mouth, this defileth a man. Matthew 15:11 KJV

August 25, _____ Day Start _____ End _____

My Prayer Focus _____

_____

Steward of My Spirit Man _____

_____

Steward of My Temple _____

_____

Steward of My Gifts _____

_____

Today I R.U.L.E. over My Life through:

Revelation	
Understanding	
Love	
Empowerment	

Exercise	
Nutrition	
Journal Notes	
Sealant	

He that believeth on me, as the scripture hath said, out of his belly shall flow rivers of living water. John 7:38 KJV

August 26, _____ Day Start _____ End _____

My Prayer Focus _____

_____

Steward of My Spirit Man _____

_____

Steward of My Temple _____

_____

Steward of My Gifts _____

_____

Today I R.U.L.E. over My Life through:

Revelation	
Understanding	
Love	
Empowerment	

Exercise	
Nutrition	
Journal Notes	
Sealant	

August 27, _____ Day Start _____ End _____

My Prayer Focus _____

_____

Steward of My Spirit Man _____

_____

Steward of My Temple _____

_____

Steward of My Gifts _____

_____

Today I R.U.L.E. over My Life through:

Revelation	
Understanding	
Love	
Empowerment	

Exercise		
Nutrition		
Journal Notes		
Sealant		

August 28, _____ Day Start _____ End _____

My Prayer Focus _____

_____

Steward of My Spirit Man _____

_____

Steward of My Temple _____

_____

Steward of My Gifts _____

_____

Today I R.U.L.E. over My Life through:

Revelation	
Understanding	
Love	
Empowerment	

Exercise	
Nutrition	
Journal Notes	
Sealant	

August 29, _____ Day Start _____ End _____

My Prayer Focus _____

_____

Steward of My Spirit Man _____

_____

Steward of My Temple _____

_____

Steward of My Gifts _____

_____

Today I R.U.L.E. over My Life through:

Revelation	
Understanding	
Love	
Empowerment	

Exercise		
Nutrition		
Journal Notes		
Sealant		

August 30, _____ Day Start _____ End _____

My Prayer Focus _____

_____

Steward of My Spirit Man _____

_____

Steward of My Temple _____

_____

Steward of My Gifts _____

_____

Today I R.U.L.E. over My Life through:

Revelation	
Understanding	
Love	
Empowerment	

Exercise	
Nutrition	
Journal Notes	
Sealant	

Consider her ways...Provides her food in the summer and gathers her supplies in the harvest. Proverbs 6:6-8

SEPTEMBER

"[After all] the kingdom of God is not a matter of [getting the] food and drink [one likes], but instead it is righteousness (that state which makes a person acceptable to God) and [heart] peace and joy in the Holy Spirit."

Romans 14:17

September 1, _____ Day Start _____ End _____

My Prayer Focus _____

_____

Steward of My Spirit Man _____

_____

Steward of My Temple _____

_____

Steward of My Gifts _____

_____

Today I R.U.L.E. over My Life through:

Revelation	
Understanding	
Love	
Empowerment	

Exercise	
Nutrition	
Journal Notes	
Sealant	

The mouth of the [uncompromisingly] righteous man is a well of life, but the mouth of the wicked conceals violence. Proverbs 10:11

September 2, ___ Day Start ____ End ___

My Prayer Focus _____

_____

Steward of My Spirit Man _____

_____

Steward of My Temple _____

_____

Steward of My Gifts _____

_____

Today I R.U.L.E. over My Life through:

Revelation	
Understanding	
Love	
Empowerment	

Exercise	
Nutrition	
Journal Notes	
Sealant	

The earnest (heartfelt, continued) prayer of a righteous man makes tremendous power available...James 5:16

September 3, ___ Day Start ____ End ___

My Prayer Focus _____

_____

Steward of My Spirit Man _____

_____

Steward of My Temple _____

_____

Steward of My Gifts _____

_____

Today I R.U.L.E. over My Life through:

Revelation	
Understanding	
Love	
Empowerment	

Exercise	
Nutrition	
Journal Notes	
Sealant	

He who receives and welcomes and accepts a righteous man ... shall receive a righteous man's reward. Matthew 10:41

September 4, ____ Day Start ____ End ____

My Prayer Focus _____

_____

Steward of My Spirit Man _____

_____

Steward of My Temple _____

_____

Steward of My Gifts _____

_____

Today I R.U.L.E. over My Life through:

Revelation	
Understanding	
Love	
Empowerment	

Exercise	
Nutrition	
Journal Notes	
Sealant	

Surely there is a reward for the [uncompromisingly] righteous; surely there is a God Who judges on the earth. Psalm 58:11

September 5, ___ Day Start ____ End ___

My Prayer Focus _____

_____

Steward of My Spirit Man _____

_____

Steward of My Temple _____

_____

Steward of My Gifts _____

_____

Today I R.U.L.E. over My Life through:

Revelation	
Understanding	
Love	
Empowerment	

Exercise	
Nutrition	
Journal Notes	
Sealant	

He who sows righteousness (moral and spiritual rectitude in every area and relation) shall have a sure reward. Proverbs 11:18

September 6, ___ Day Start ____ End ___

My Prayer Focus _____

_____

Steward of My Spirit Man _____

_____

Steward of My Temple _____

_____

Steward of My Gifts _____

_____

Today I R.U.L.E. over My Life through:

Revelation	
Understanding	
Love	
Empowerment	

Exercise	
Nutrition	
Journal Notes	
Sealant	

September 7, ____ Day Start ____ End ____

My Prayer Focus _____
_____

Steward of My Spirit Man _____
_____

Steward of My Temple _____
_____

Steward of My Gifts _____
_____

Today I R.U.L.E. over My Life through:

Revelation	
Understanding	
Love	
Empowerment	

Exercise	
Nutrition	
Journal Notes	
Sealant	

September 8, _____ Day Start _____ End _____

My Prayer Focus _____

_____

Steward of My Spirit Man _____

_____

Steward of My Temple _____

_____

Steward of My Gifts _____

_____

Today I R.U.L.E. over My Life through:

Revelation	
Understanding	
Love	
Empowerment	

Exercise	
Nutrition	
Journal Notes	
Sealant	

September 9, _____ Day Start _____ End _____

My Prayer Focus _____

_____

Steward of My Spirit Man _____

_____

Steward of My Temple _____

_____

Steward of My Gifts _____

_____

Today I R.U.L.E. over My Life through:

Revelation	
Understanding	
Love	
Empowerment	

Exercise	
Nutrition	
Journal Notes	
Sealant	

September 10,___ Day Start ____ End ___

My Prayer Focus _____

_____

Steward of My Spirit Man _____

_____

Steward of My Temple _____

_____

Steward of My Gifts _____

_____

Today I R.U.L.E. over My Life through:

Revelation	
Understanding	
Love	
Empowerment	

Exercise	
Nutrition	
Journal Notes	
Sealant	

September 11,____ Day Start _____ End ____

My Prayer Focus _____

_____

Steward of My Spirit Man _____

_____

Steward of My Temple _____

_____

Steward of My Gifts _____

_____

Today I R.U.L.E. over My Life through:

Revelation	
Understanding	
Love	
Empowerment	

Exercise	
Nutrition	
Journal Notes	
Sealant	

When the righteous cry for help, the Lord hears, and delivers them out of all their distress and troubles. Psalm 34:17

September 12,____ Day Start _____ End ____

My Prayer Focus _____

_____

Steward of My Spirit Man _____

_____

Steward of My Temple _____

_____

Steward of My Gifts _____

_____

Today I R.U.L.E. over My Life through:

Revelation	
Understanding	
Love	
Empowerment	

Exercise	
Nutrition	
Journal Notes	
Sealant	

September 13,____ Day Start _____ End ____

My Prayer Focus _____

_____

Steward of My Spirit Man _____

_____

Steward of My Temple _____

_____

Steward of My Gifts _____

_____

Today I R.U.L.E. over My Life through:

Revelation	
Understanding	
Love	
Empowerment	

Exercise	
Nutrition	
Journal Notes	
Sealant	

He will never allow the [consistently] righteous to be moved (made to slip, fall, or fail). Psalm 55:22

September 14,___ Day Start ____ End ___

My Prayer Focus _____

_____

Steward of My Spirit Man _____

_____

Steward of My Temple _____

_____

Steward of My Gifts _____

_____

Today I R.U.L.E. over My Life through:

Revelation	
Understanding	
Love	
Empowerment	

Exercise	
Nutrition	
Journal Notes	
Sealant	

September 15,____ Day Start _____ End ____

My Prayer Focus _____

_____

Steward of My Spirit Man _____

_____

Steward of My Temple _____

_____

Steward of My Gifts _____

_____

Today I R.U.L.E. over My Life through:

Revelation	
Understanding	
Love	
Empowerment	

Exercise	
Nutrition	
Journal Notes	
Sealant	

The Lord is far from the wicked, but He hears the prayer of the [consistently] righteous (the upright...). Proverbs 15:29

September 16,___ Day Start _____ End ___

My Prayer Focus _____

_____

Steward of My Spirit Man _____

_____

Steward of My Temple _____

_____

Steward of My Gifts _____

_____

Today I R.U.L.E. over My Life through:

Revelation	
Understanding	
Love	
Empowerment	

Exercise		
Nutrition		
Journal Notes		
Sealant		

Better is the little that the [uncompromisingly] righteous have than the abundance...of many who are...wicked. Psalm 37:16

September 17,____ Day Start ____ End ____

My Prayer Focus _____

_____

Steward of My Spirit Man _____

_____

Steward of My Temple _____

_____

Steward of My Gifts _____

_____

Today I R.U.L.E. over My Life through:

Revelation	
Understanding	
Love	
Empowerment	

Exercise	
Nutrition	
Journal Notes	
Sealant	

Blessed are they which do hunger and thirst after righteousness: for they shall be filled. Matthew 5:6 KJV

September 18,___ Day Start ____ End ___

My Prayer Focus _____

Steward of My Spirit Man _____

Steward of My Temple _____

Steward of My Gifts _____

Today I R.U.L.E. over My Life through:

Revelation	
Understanding	
Love	
Empowerment	

Exercise	
Nutrition	
Journal Notes	
Sealant	

September 19,_____ Day Start _____ End _____

My Prayer Focus _____

_____

Steward of My Spirit Man _____

_____

Steward of My Temple _____

_____

Steward of My Gifts _____

_____

Today I R.U.L.E. over My Life through:

Revelation	
Understanding	
Love	
Empowerment	

Exercise	
Nutrition	
Journal Notes	
Sealant	

You shall establish yourself in righteousness (rightness, in conformity with God's will and order). Isaiah 54:14

September 20,___ Day Start ____ End ___

My Prayer Focus _____

_____

Steward of My Spirit Man _____

_____

Steward of My Temple _____

_____

Steward of My Gifts _____

_____

Today I R.U.L.E. over My Life through:

Revelation	
Understanding	
Love	
Empowerment	

Exercise	
Nutrition	
Journal Notes	
Sealant	

September 21,____ Day Start _____ End ____

My Prayer Focus _____

_____

Steward of My Spirit Man _____

_____

Steward of My Temple _____

_____

Steward of My Gifts _____

_____

Today I R.U.L.E. over My Life through:

Revelation	
Understanding	
Love	
Empowerment	

Exercise	
Nutrition	
Journal Notes	
Sealant	

September 22,____ Day Start _____ End ___

My Prayer Focus _____

_____

Steward of My Spirit Man _____

_____

Steward of My Temple _____

_____

Steward of My Gifts _____

_____

Today I R.U.L.E. over My Life through:

Revelation	
Understanding	
Love	
Empowerment	

Exercise	
Nutrition	
Journal Notes	
Sealant	

Unless your righteousness (your uprightness and your right standing with God) is more than that of the scribes...Matthew 5:20

September 23,_____ Day Start _____ End _____

My Prayer Focus _____

_____

Steward of My Spirit Man _____

_____

Steward of My Temple _____

_____

Steward of My Gifts _____

_____

Today I R.U.L.E. over My Life through:

Revelation	
Understanding	
Love	
Empowerment	

Exercise	
Nutrition	
Journal Notes	
Sealant	

September 24,____ Day Start _____ End ____

My Prayer Focus _____

_____

Steward of My Spirit Man _____

_____

Steward of My Temple _____

_____

Steward of My Gifts _____

_____

Today I R.U.L.E. over My Life through:

Revelation	
Understanding	
Love	
Empowerment	

Exercise	
Nutrition	
Journal Notes	
Sealant	

Hear the cases between your brethren and judge righteously ... Deuteronomy 1:16

September 25,____ Day Start _____ End ____

My Prayer Focus _____

_____

Steward of My Spirit Man _____

_____

Steward of My Temple _____

_____

Steward of My Gifts _____

_____

Today I R.U.L.E. over My Life through:

Revelation	
Understanding	
Love	
Empowerment	

Exercise	
Nutrition	
Journal Notes	
Sealant	

His own arm brought Him victory, and His own righteousness [having the Spirit without measure] sustained Him. Isaiah 59:16

September 26,____ Day Start _____ End ____

My Prayer Focus _____

_____

Steward of My Spirit Man _____

_____

Steward of My Temple _____

_____

Steward of My Gifts _____

_____

Today I R.U.L.E. over My Life through:

Revelation	
Understanding	
Love	
Empowerment	

Exercise	
Nutrition	
Journal Notes	
Sealant	

He who practices righteousness...is righteous, even as He is righteous. 1 John 3:7

September 27,____ Day Start _____ End ____

My Prayer Focus _____

_____

Steward of My Spirit Man _____

_____

Steward of My Temple _____

_____

Steward of My Gifts _____

_____

Today I R.U.L.E. over My Life through:

Revelation	
Understanding	
Love	
Empowerment	

Exercise		
Nutrition		
Journal Notes		
Sealant		

September 28,___ Day Start _____ End ___

My Prayer Focus _____

_____

Steward of My Spirit Man _____

_____

Steward of My Temple _____

_____

Steward of My Gifts _____

_____

Today I R.U.L.E. over My Life through:

Revelation	
Understanding	
Love	
Empowerment	

Exercise	
Nutrition	
Journal Notes	
Sealant	

Through Him we might become...the righteousness of God. 2 Corinthians 5:21

September 29,____ Day Start ____ End ____

My Prayer Focus _____

_____

Steward of My Spirit Man _____

_____

Steward of My Temple _____

_____

Steward of My Gifts _____

_____

Today I R.U.L.E. over My Life through:

Revelation	
Understanding	
Love	
Empowerment	

Exercise	
Nutrition	
Journal Notes	
Sealant	

September 30,____ Day Start _____ End ____

My Prayer Focus _____

_____

Steward of My Spirit Man _____

_____

Steward of My Temple _____

_____

Steward of My Gifts _____

_____

Today I R.U.L.E. over My Life through:

Revelation	
Understanding	
Love	
Empowerment	

Exercise	
Nutrition	
Journal Notes	
Sealant	

EMPOWERMENT

RULE No. 4

I MUST FIGHT KNOWING THAT I HAVE ALREADY WON

I looked [them over] and rose up and said to the nobles and officials and the other people, Do not be afraid of the enemy; [earnestly] remember the Lord and imprint Him [on your minds], great and terrible, and [take from Him courage to] fight for your brethren, your sons, your daughters, your wives, and your homes. And when our enemies heard that their plot was known to us and that God had frustrated their purpose, we all returned to the wall, everyone to his work.. Our God will fight for us.
Nehemiah 4:14-20

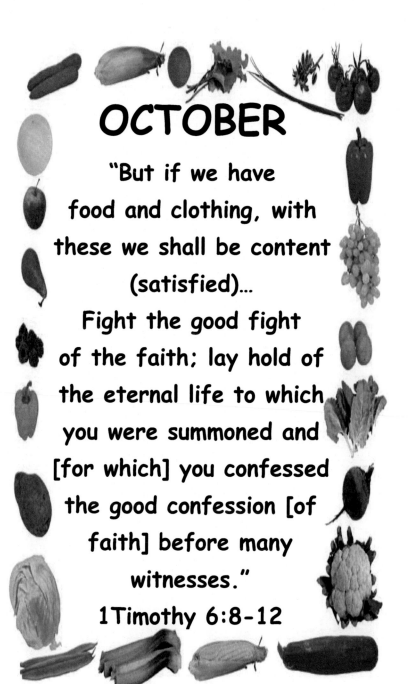

OCTOBER

"But if we have food and clothing, with these we shall be content (satisfied)...
Fight the good fight of the faith; lay hold of the eternal life to which you were summoned and [for which] you confessed the good confession [of faith] before many witnesses."
1Timothy 6:8-12

October 1, _____   Day Start _____ End ___

My Prayer Focus _____

_____

Steward of My Spirit Man _____

_____

Steward of My Temple _____

_____

Steward of My Gifts _____

_____

Today I R.U.L.E. over My Life through:

Revelation	
Understanding	
Love	
Empowerment	

Exercise	
Nutrition	
Journal Notes	
Sealant	

October 2, _____   Day Start _____ End _____

My Prayer Focus _____

_____

Steward of My Spirit Man _____

_____

Steward of My Temple _____

_____

Steward of My Gifts _____

_____

Today I R.U.L.E. over My Life through:

Revelation	
Understanding	
Love	
Empowerment	

Exercise	
Nutrition	
Journal Notes	
Sealant	

October 3, _____   Day Start _____ End _____

My Prayer Focus _____

_____

Steward of My Spirit Man _____

_____

Steward of My Temple _____

_____

Steward of My Gifts _____

_____

Today I R.U.L.E. over My Life through:

Revelation	
Understanding	
Love	
Empowerment	

Exercise	
Nutrition	
Journal Notes	
Sealant	

October 4, _____   Day Start _____ End _____

My Prayer Focus _____

_____

Steward of My Spirit Man _____

_____

Steward of My Temple _____

_____

Steward of My Gifts _____

_____

Today I R.U.L.E. over My Life through:

Revelation	
Understanding	
Love	
Empowerment	

Exercise	
Nutrition	
Journal Notes	
Sealant	

Now faith is the assurance (the confirmation, the title deed) of the things [we] hope for...Hebrews 11:1

October 5, _____   Day Start _____ End _____

My Prayer Focus _____

_____

Steward of My Spirit Man _____

_____

Steward of My Temple _____

_____

Steward of My Gifts _____

_____

Today I R.U.L.E. over My Life through:

Revelation	
Understanding	
Love	
Empowerment	

Exercise	
Nutrition	
Journal Notes	
Sealant	

October 6, _____   Day Start _____   End _____

My Prayer Focus _____

_____

Steward of My Spirit Man _____

_____

Steward of My Temple _____

_____

Steward of My Gifts _____

_____

Today I R.U.L.E. over My Life through:

Revelation	
Understanding	
Love	
Empowerment	

Exercise	
Nutrition	
Journal Notes	
Sealant	

The man who through faith is just and upright shall live and shall live by faith. Romans 1:17

October 7, _____ Day Start _____ End _____

My Prayer Focus _____

_____

Steward of My Spirit Man _____

_____

Steward of My Temple _____

_____

Steward of My Gifts _____

_____

Today I R.U.L.E. over My Life through:

Revelation	
Understanding	
Love	
Empowerment	

Exercise	
Nutrition	
Journal Notes	
Sealant	

October 8, _____   Day Start _____   End _____

My Prayer Focus _____

_____

Steward of My Spirit Man _____

_____

Steward of My Temple _____

_____

Steward of My Gifts _____

_____

Today I R.U.L.E. over My Life through:

Revelation	
Understanding	
Love	
Empowerment	

Exercise	
Nutrition	
Journal Notes	
Sealant	

If you had faith (trust and confidence in God) even [so small] like a grain of mustard seed...Luke 17:6

October 9, _____   Day Start _____ End _____

My Prayer Focus _____

_____

Steward of My Spirit Man _____

_____

Steward of My Temple _____

_____

Steward of My Gifts _____

_____

Today I R.U.L.E. over My Life through:

Revelation	
Understanding	
Love	
Empowerment	

Exercise	
Nutrition	
Journal Notes	
Sealant	

Take courage, daughter your faith has made you well. And at once the woman was restored to health. Matthew 9:22

October 10,_____   Day Start _____ End ____

My Prayer Focus _____

_____

Steward of My Spirit Man _____

_____

Steward of My Temple _____

_____

Steward of My Gifts _____

_____

Today I R.U.L.E. over My Life through:

Revelation	
Understanding	
Love	
Empowerment	

Exercise	
Nutrition	
Journal Notes	
Sealant	

And so faith, hope, love abide [faith--conviction and belief respecting man's relation to God and divine things...1 Corinthians 13:13

October 11,_____ Day Start _____ End _____

My Prayer Focus _____

_____

Steward of My Spirit Man _____

_____

Steward of My Temple _____

_____

Steward of My Gifts _____

_____

Today I R.U.L.E. over My Life through:

Revelation	
Understanding	
Love	
Empowerment	

Exercise	
Nutrition	
Journal Notes	
Sealant	

So also faith, if it does not have works (deeds and actions of obedience to back it up), by itself is destitute of power. James 2:17

October 12,_____   Day Start _____ End _____

My Prayer Focus _____

_____

Steward of My Spirit Man _____

_____

Steward of My Temple _____

_____

Steward of My Gifts _____

_____

Today I R.U.L.E. over My Life through:

Revelation	
Understanding	
Love	
Empowerment	

Exercise	
Nutrition	
Journal Notes	
Sealant	

October 13,_____   Day Start _____ End ____

My Prayer Focus _____

_____

Steward of My Spirit Man _____

_____

Steward of My Temple _____

_____

Steward of My Gifts _____

_____

Today I R.U.L.E. over My Life through:

Revelation	
Understanding	
Love	
Empowerment	

Exercise	
Nutrition	
Journal Notes	
Sealant	

October 14,_____ Day Start _____ End ____

My Prayer Focus _____

_____

Steward of My Spirit Man _____

_____

Steward of My Temple _____

_____

Steward of My Gifts _____

_____

Today I R.U.L.E. over My Life through:

Revelation	
Understanding	
Love	
Empowerment	

Exercise		
Nutrition		
Journal Notes		
Sealant		

You have been faithful and trustworthy over a little; I will put you in charge of much. Matthew 25:21

October 15,_____   Day Start _____ End _____

My Prayer Focus _____

_____

Steward of My Spirit Man _____

_____

Steward of My Temple _____

_____

Steward of My Gifts _____

_____

Today I R.U.L.E. over My Life through:

Revelation	
Understanding	
Love	
Empowerment	

Exercise	
Nutrition	
Journal Notes	
Sealant	

October 16,_____   Day Start _____ End _____

My Prayer Focus _____

_____

Steward of My Spirit Man _____

_____

Steward of My Temple _____

_____

Steward of My Gifts _____

_____

Today I R.U.L.E. over My Life through:

Revelation	
Understanding	
Love	
Empowerment	

Exercise	
Nutrition	
Journal Notes	
Sealant	

The Lord will fight for you, and you shall hold your peace and remain at rest. Exodus 14:14

October 17,_____   Day Start _____ End _____

My Prayer Focus _____

_____

Steward of My Spirit Man _____

_____

Steward of My Temple _____

_____

Steward of My Gifts _____

_____

Today I R.U.L.E. over My Life through:

Revelation	
Understanding	
Love	
Empowerment	

Exercise		
Nutrition		
Journal Notes		
Sealant		

One man of you shall put to flight a thousand, for it is the Lord your God Who fights for you, as He promised you. Joshua 23:10

October 18,_____   Day Start _____ End ___

My Prayer Focus _____

_____

Steward of My Spirit Man _____

_____

Steward of My Temple _____

_____

Steward of My Gifts _____

_____

Today I R.U.L.E. over My Life through:

Revelation	
Understanding	
Love	
Empowerment	

Exercise	
Nutrition	
Journal Notes	
Sealant	

Let no man's heart fail because of this Philistine; your servant will go out and fight with him. 1 Samuel 17:32

October 19,_____ Day Start _____ End _____

My Prayer Focus _____

_____

Steward of My Spirit Man _____

_____

Steward of My Temple _____

_____

Steward of My Gifts _____

_____

Today I R.U.L.E. over My Life through:

Revelation	
Understanding	
Love	
Empowerment	

Exercise	
Nutrition	
Journal Notes	
Sealant	

Choose us out men and go out, fight with Amalek...I will stand on the top of the hill with the rod of God in my hand. Exodus 17:9

October 20,_____   Day Start _____ End _____

My Prayer Focus _____

_____

Steward of My Spirit Man _____

_____

Steward of My Temple _____

_____

Steward of My Gifts _____

_____

Today I R.U.L.E. over My Life through:

Revelation	
Understanding	
Love	
Empowerment	

Exercise	
Nutrition	
Journal Notes	
Sealant	

I have fought a good fight, I have finished my course, I have kept the faith. 2 Timothy 4:7 KJV

October 21,_____   Day Start _____ End _____

My Prayer Focus _____

_____

Steward of My Spirit Man _____

_____

Steward of My Temple _____

_____

Steward of My Gifts _____

_____

Today I R.U.L.E. over My Life through:

Revelation	
Understanding	
Love	
Empowerment	

Exercise	
Nutrition	
Journal Notes	
Sealant	

There was no day like it before or since, when the Lord heeded the voice of a man. For the Lord fought for Israel. Joshua 10:14

October 22,_____   Day Start _____ End _____

My Prayer Focus _____

_____

Steward of My Spirit Man _____

_____

Steward of My Temple _____

_____

Steward of My Gifts _____

_____

Today I R.U.L.E. over My Life through:

Revelation	
Understanding	
Love	
Empowerment	

Exercise	
Nutrition	
Journal Notes	
Sealant	

October 23,_____   Day Start _____ End _____

My Prayer Focus _____

_____

Steward of My Spirit Man _____

_____

Steward of My Temple _____

_____

Steward of My Gifts _____

_____

Today I R.U.L.E. over My Life through:

Revelation	
Understanding	
Love	
Empowerment	

Exercise	
Nutrition	
Journal Notes	
Sealant	

They cried to God in the battle...He granted their entreaty... they relied on, clung to, and trusted in Him. 1 Chronicles 5:20

October 24,____   Day Start ____   End ___

My Prayer Focus _____

_____

Steward of My Spirit Man _____

_____

Steward of My Temple _____

_____

Steward of My Gifts _____

_____

Today I R.U.L.E. over My Life through:

Revelation	
Understanding	
Love	
Empowerment	

Exercise	
Nutrition	
Journal Notes	
Sealant	

With him is an arm of flesh, but with us is the Lord our God to help us and to fight our battles. 2 Chronicles 32:8

October 25,_____   Day Start _____ End ___

My Prayer Focus _____

_____

Steward of My Spirit Man _____

_____

Steward of My Temple _____

_____

Steward of My Gifts _____

_____

Today I R.U.L.E. over My Life through:

Revelation	
Understanding	
Love	
Empowerment	

Exercise	
Nutrition	
Journal Notes	
Sealant	

Who is the King of glory? The Lord strong and mighty, the Lord mighty in battle. Psalm 24:8

October 26,_____ Day Start _____ End _____

My Prayer Focus _____

_____

Steward of My Spirit Man _____

_____

Steward of My Temple _____

_____

Steward of My Gifts _____

_____

Today I R.U.L.E. over My Life through:

Revelation	
Understanding	
Love	
Empowerment	

Exercise	
Nutrition	
Journal Notes	
Sealant	

But I have prayed for thee, that thy faith fail not. Luke 22:32 KJV

October 27,_____   Day Start _____ End ___

My Prayer Focus _____

_____

Steward of My Spirit Man _____

_____

Steward of My Temple _____

_____

Steward of My Gifts _____

_____

Today I R.U.L.E. over My Life through:

Revelation	
Understanding	
Love	
Empowerment	

Exercise	
Nutrition	
Journal Notes	
Sealant	

God is faithful, by whom ye were called unto the fellowship of his Son Jesus Christ our Lord. 1 Corinthians 1:9 KJV

October 28,_____ Day Start _____ End _____

My Prayer Focus _____

_____

Steward of My Spirit Man _____

_____

Steward of My Temple _____

_____

Steward of My Gifts _____

_____

Today I R.U.L.E. over My Life through:

Revelation	
Understanding	
Love	
Empowerment	

Exercise	
Nutrition	
Journal Notes	
Sealant	

October 29,_____   Day Start _____ End _____

My Prayer Focus _____

_____

Steward of My Spirit Man _____

_____

Steward of My Temple _____

_____

Steward of My Gifts _____

_____

Today I R.U.L.E. over My Life through:

Revelation	
Understanding	
Love	
Empowerment	

Exercise	
Nutrition	
Journal Notes	
Sealant	

Through faith subdued kingdoms, wrought righteousness, obtained promises, stopped the mouths of lions Hebrews 11:33

October 30,_____   Day Start _____ End _____

My Prayer Focus _____

_____

Steward of My Spirit Man _____

_____

Steward of My Temple _____

_____

Steward of My Gifts _____

_____

Today I R.U.L.E. over My Life through:

Revelation	
Understanding	
Love	
Empowerment	

Exercise	
Nutrition	
Journal Notes	
Sealant	

If ye continue in the faith grounded and settled and be not moved away from the hope of the gospel. Colossians 1:23 KJV

October 31,_____   Day Start _____ End _____

My Prayer Focus _____

_____

Steward of My Spirit Man _____

_____

Steward of My Temple _____

_____

Steward of My Gifts _____

_____

Today I R.U.L.E. over My Life through:

Revelation	
Understanding	
Love	
Empowerment	

Exercise	
Nutrition	
Journal Notes	
Sealant	

Looking unto Jesus the author and finisher of our faith...Hebrews 12:2 KJV

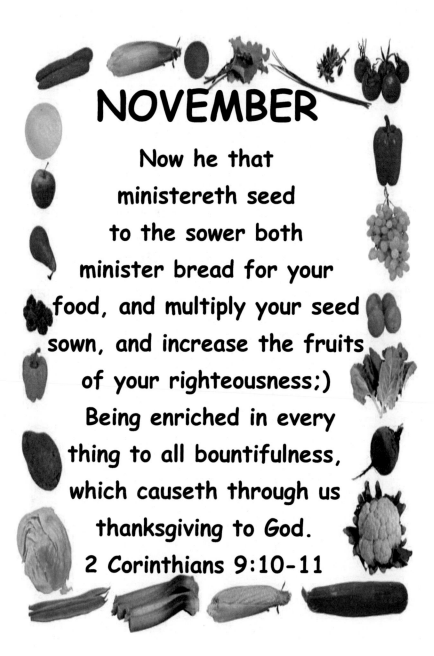

NOVEMBER

Now he that
ministereth seed
to the sower both
minister bread for your
food, and multiply your seed
sown, and increase the fruits
of your righteousness;)
Being enriched in every
thing to all bountifulness,
which causeth through us
thanksgiving to God.
2 Corinthians 9:10-11

November 1, ____ Day Start _____ End ____

My Prayer Focus _____

_____

Steward of My Spirit Man _____

_____

Steward of My Temple _____

_____

Steward of My Gifts _____

_____

Today I R.U.L.E. over My Life through:

Revelation	
Understanding	
Love	
Empowerment	

Exercise	
Nutrition	
Journal Notes	
Sealant	

It has been written, Man shall not live and be upheld and sustained by br.ead alone...Mathew 4:4

November 2, ___ Day Start ____ End ___

My Prayer Focus _____

_____

Steward of My Spirit Man _____

_____

Steward of My Temple _____

_____

Steward of My Gifts _____

_____

Today I R.U.L.E. over My Life through:

Revelation	
Understanding	
Love	
Empowerment	

Exercise	
Nutrition	
Journal Notes	
Sealant	

November 3, ____ Day Start ____ End ____

My Prayer Focus _____

_____

Steward of My Spirit Man _____

_____

Steward of My Temple _____

_____

Steward of My Gifts _____

_____

Today I R.U.L.E. over My Life through:

Revelation	
Understanding	
Love	
Empowerment	

Exercise	
Nutrition	
Journal Notes	
Sealant	

November 4, ____ Day Start _____ End ____

My Prayer Focus _____

_____

Steward of My Spirit Man _____

_____

Steward of My Temple _____

_____

Steward of My Gifts _____

_____

Today I R.U.L.E. over My Life through:

Revelation	
Understanding	
Love	
Empowerment	

Exercise	
Nutrition	
Journal Notes	
Sealant	

For the Word that God speaks is alive and full of power [making it active, operative, energizing, and effective]...Hebrews 4:12

November 5, _____ Day Start _____ End _____

My Prayer Focus _____

_____

Steward of My Spirit Man _____

_____

Steward of My Temple _____

_____

Steward of My Gifts _____

_____

Today I R.U.L.E. over My Life through:

Revelation	
Understanding	
Love	
Empowerment	

Exercise	
Nutrition	
Journal Notes	
Sealant	

Sanctify them [purify, consecrate, separate them for Yourself, make them holy] by the Truth; Your Word is Truth. John 17:17

November 6, ___ Day Start ____ End ___

My Prayer Focus _____

_____

Steward of My Spirit Man _____

_____

Steward of My Temple _____

_____

Steward of My Gifts _____

_____

Today I R.U.L.E. over My Life through:

Revelation	
Understanding	
Love	
Empowerment	

Exercise		
Nutrition		
Journal Notes		
Sealant		

The word is nigh thee, even in thy mouth, and in thy heart: that is, the word of faith, which we preach...Romans 10:8

November 7, ___ Day Start ____ End ___

My Prayer Focus _____

_____

Steward of My Spirit Man _____

_____

Steward of My Temple _____

_____

Steward of My Gifts _____

_____

Today I R.U.L.E. over My Life through:

Revelation	
Understanding	
Love	
Empowerment	

Exercise	
Nutrition	
Journal Notes	
Sealant	

November 8, ____ Day Start ____ End ____

My Prayer Focus _____

_____

Steward of My Spirit Man _____

_____

Steward of My Temple _____

_____

Steward of My Gifts _____

_____

Today I R.U.L.E. over My Life through:

Revelation	
Understanding	
Love	
Empowerment	

Exercise	
Nutrition	
Journal Notes	
Sealant	

It is the spirit that quickeneth...flesh profiteth nothing: the words that I speak unto you, they are spirit, and ... life. John 6:63 KJV

November 9, _____ Day Start _____ End _____

My Prayer Focus _____

_____

Steward of My Spirit Man _____

_____

Steward of My Temple _____

_____

Steward of My Gifts _____

_____

Today I R.U.L.E. over My Life through:

Revelation	
Understanding	
Love	
Empowerment	

Exercise	
Nutrition	
Journal Notes	
Sealant	

And they were amazed at His teaching, for His word was with authority and ability and weight and power. Luke 4:32

November 10,____ Day Start _____ End ____

My Prayer Focus _____

_____

Steward of My Spirit Man _____

_____

Steward of My Temple _____

_____

Steward of My Gifts _____

_____

Today I R.U.L.E. over My Life through:

Revelation	
Understanding	
Love	
Empowerment	

Exercise	
Nutrition	
Journal Notes	
Sealant	

Because thou hast kept the word of my patience, I also will keep thee from the hour of temptation. Revelation 3:10 KJV

November 11,____ Day Start _____ End ____

My Prayer Focus _____

_____

Steward of My Spirit Man _____

_____

Steward of My Temple _____

_____

Steward of My Gifts _____

_____

Today I R.U.L.E. over My Life through:

Revelation	
Understanding	
Love	
Empowerment	

Exercise	
Nutrition	
Journal Notes	
Sealant	

Through faith we understand that the worlds were framed by the word of God...Hebrews 11:3

November 12,_____ Day Start _____ End _____

My Prayer Focus _____

_____

Steward of My Spirit Man _____

_____

Steward of My Temple _____

_____

Steward of My Gifts _____

_____

Today I R.U.L.E. over My Life through:

Revelation	
Understanding	
Love	
Empowerment	

Exercise	
Nutrition	
Journal Notes	
Sealant	

November 13,____ Day Start _____ End ____

My Prayer Focus _____

_____

Steward of My Spirit Man _____

_____

Steward of My Temple _____

_____

Steward of My Gifts _____

_____

Today I R.U.L.E. over My Life through:

Revelation	
Understanding	
Love	
Empowerment	

Exercise	
Nutrition	
Journal Notes	
Sealant	

You are nullifying and making void and of no effect [the authority of] the Word of God through your tradition.... Mark 7:13

November 14,____ Day Start _____ End ____

My Prayer Focus _____

_____

Steward of My Spirit Man _____

_____

Steward of My Temple _____

_____

Steward of My Gifts _____

_____

Today I R.U.L.E. over My Life through:

Revelation	
Understanding	
Love	
Empowerment	

Exercise	
Nutrition	
Journal Notes	
Sealant	

Order my steps in thy word: and let not any iniquity have dominion over me. Psalm 119:133 KJV

November 15,____ Day Start _____ End ____

My Prayer Focus _____

_____

Steward of My Spirit Man _____

_____

Steward of My Temple _____

_____

Steward of My Gifts _____

_____

Today I R.U.L.E. over My Life through:

Revelation	
Understanding	
Love	
Empowerment	

Exercise	
Nutrition	
Journal Notes	
Sealant	

November 16,____ Day Start ____ End ____

My Prayer Focus _____

_____

Steward of My Spirit Man _____

_____

Steward of My Temple _____

_____

Steward of My Gifts _____

_____

Today I R.U.L.E. over My Life through:

Revelation	
Understanding	
Love	
Empowerment	

Exercise	
Nutrition	
Journal Notes	
Sealant	

It shall accomplish that which I please and purpose, and it shall prosper...Isaiah 55:11

November 17,_____ Day Start _____ End _____

My Prayer Focus _____

_____

Steward of My Spirit Man _____

_____

Steward of My Temple _____

_____

Steward of My Gifts _____

_____

Today I R.U.L.E. over My Life through:

Revelation	
Understanding	
Love	
Empowerment	

Exercise	
Nutrition	
Journal Notes	
Sealant	

A word fitly spoken and in due season is like apples of gold in settings of silver. Proverbs 25:11

November 18,____ Day Start _____ End ____

My Prayer Focus _____

_____

Steward of My Spirit Man _____

_____

Steward of My Temple _____

_____

Steward of My Gifts _____

_____

Today I R.U.L.E. over My Life through:

Revelation	
Understanding	
Love	
Empowerment	

Exercise	
Nutrition	
Journal Notes	
Sealant	

Princes pursue and persecute me without cause, but my heart stands in awe of Your words. Psalm 119:161

November 19,____ Day Start _____ End ___

My Prayer Focus _____

_____

Steward of My Spirit Man _____

_____

Steward of My Temple _____

_____

Steward of My Gifts _____

_____

Today I R.U.L.E. over My Life through:

Revelation	
Understanding	
Love	
Empowerment	

Exercise	
Nutrition	
Journal Notes	
Sealant	

Hear [O Jerusalem] the word of the Lord, you rulers or judges. Isaiah 1:10

November 20,____ Day Start ____ End ____

My Prayer Focus _____

_____

Steward of My Spirit Man _____

_____

Steward of My Temple _____

_____

Steward of My Gifts _____

_____

Today I R.U.L.E. over My Life through:

Revelation	
Understanding	
Love	
Empowerment	

Exercise	
Nutrition	
Journal Notes	
Sealant	

November 21,____ Day Start _____ End ____

My Prayer Focus _____

_____

Steward of My Spirit Man _____

_____

Steward of My Temple _____

_____

Steward of My Gifts _____

_____

Today I R.U.L.E. over My Life through:

Revelation	
Understanding	
Love	
Empowerment	

Exercise		
Nutrition		
Journal Notes		
Sealant		

November 22,____ Day Start _____ End ____

My Prayer Focus _____

_____

Steward of My Spirit Man _____

_____

Steward of My Temple _____

_____

Steward of My Gifts _____

_____

Today I R.U.L.E. over My Life through:

Revelation	
Understanding	
Love	
Empowerment	

Exercise	
Nutrition	
Journal Notes	
Sealant	

And have felt how good the Word of God is and the mighty powers of the age and world to come. Hebrews 6:5

November 23,____ Day Start _____ End ____

My Prayer Focus _____

_____

Steward of My Spirit Man _____

_____

Steward of My Temple _____

_____

Steward of My Gifts _____

_____

Today I R.U.L.E. over My Life through:

Revelation	
Understanding	
Love	
Empowerment	

Exercise	
Nutrition	
Journal Notes	
Sealant	

November 24,____ Day Start _____ End ____

My Prayer Focus _____

_____

Steward of My Spirit Man _____

_____

Steward of My Temple _____

_____

Steward of My Gifts _____

_____

Today I R.U.L.E. over My Life through:

Revelation	
Understanding	
Love	
Empowerment	

Exercise	
Nutrition	
Journal Notes	
Sealant	

But we will continue to devote ourselves steadfastly to prayer and the ministry of the Word. Acts 6:4

November 25,___ Day Start ____ End ___

My Prayer Focus _____

_____

Steward of My Spirit Man _____

_____

Steward of My Temple _____

_____

Steward of My Gifts _____

_____

Today I R.U.L.E. over My Life through:

Revelation	
Understanding	
Love	
Empowerment	

Exercise	
Nutrition	
Journal Notes	
Sealant	

Let the words of my mouth, and the meditation of my heart, be acceptable in thy sight, O LORD... my redeemer. Psalm 19:14

November 26,____ Day Start _____ End ____

My Prayer Focus _____

_____

Steward of My Spirit Man _____

_____

Steward of My Temple _____

_____

Steward of My Gifts _____

_____

Today I R.U.L.E. over My Life through:

Revelation	
Understanding	
Love	
Empowerment	

Exercise	
Nutrition	
Journal Notes	
Sealant	

My son, keep my words; lay up within you my commandments [for use when needed] and treasure them. Proverbs 7:1

November 27,___ Day Start ____ End ___

My Prayer Focus _____
_____

Steward of My Spirit Man _____
_____

Steward of My Temple _____
_____

Steward of My Gifts _____
_____

Today I R.U.L.E. over My Life through:

Revelation	
Understanding	
Love	
Empowerment	

Exercise	
Nutrition	
Journal Notes	
Sealant	

He that is of God heareth God's words: ye therefore hear them not, because ye are not of God. John 8:47 KJV

November 28,____ Day Start _____ End ____

My Prayer Focus _____

_____

Steward of My Spirit Man _____

_____

Steward of My Temple _____

_____

Steward of My Gifts _____

_____

Today I R.U.L.E. over My Life through:

Revelation	
Understanding	
Love	
Empowerment	

Exercise	
Nutrition	
Journal Notes	
Sealant	

November 29,____ Day Start _____ End ____

My Prayer Focus _____

_____

Steward of My Spirit Man _____

_____

Steward of My Temple _____

_____

Steward of My Gifts _____

_____

Today I R.U.L.E. over My Life through:

Revelation	
Understanding	
Love	
Empowerment	

Exercise	
Nutrition	
Journal Notes	
Sealant	

November 30,___ Day Start _____ End ___

My Prayer Focus _____

_____

Steward of My Spirit Man _____

_____

Steward of My Temple _____

_____

Steward of My Gifts _____

_____

Today I R.U.L.E. over My Life through:

Revelation	
Understanding	
Love	
Empowerment	

Exercise	
Nutrition	
Journal Notes	
Sealant	

But the word of God grew and multiplied. Acts 12:24

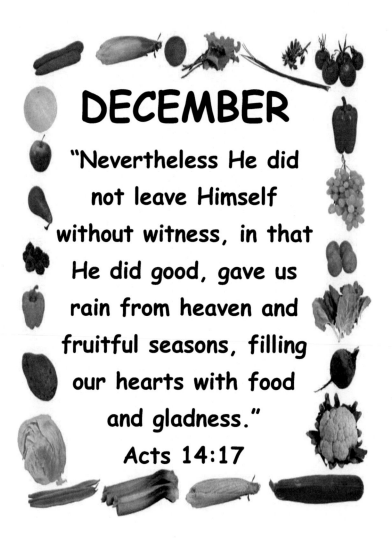

DECEMBER

"Nevertheless He did not leave Himself without witness, in that He did good, gave us rain from heaven and fruitful seasons, filling our hearts with food and gladness."

Acts 14:17

December 1, _____ Day Start _____ End _____

My Prayer Focus _____

_____

Steward of My Spirit Man _____

_____

Steward of My Temple _____

_____

Steward of My Gifts _____

_____

Today I R.U.L.E. over My Life through:

Revelation	
Understanding	
Love	
Empowerment	

Exercise		
Nutrition		
Journal Notes		
Sealant		

December 2, _____ Day Start _____ End _____

My Prayer Focus _____

_____

Steward of My Spirit Man _____

_____

Steward of My Temple _____

_____

Steward of My Gifts _____

_____

Today I R.U.L.E. over My Life through:

Revelation	
Understanding	
Love	
Empowerment	

Exercise	
Nutrition	
Journal Notes	
Sealant	

He causes to come down for you the rain, the former rain and the latter rain, as before. Joel 2:23

December 3, _____ Day Start _____ End ___

My Prayer Focus _____

_____

Steward of My Spirit Man _____

_____

Steward of My Temple _____

_____

Steward of My Gifts _____

_____

Today I R.U.L.E. over My Life through:

Revelation	
Understanding	
Love	
Empowerment	

Exercise	
Nutrition	
Journal Notes	
Sealant	

December 4, _____ Day Start _____ End _____

My Prayer Focus _____

_____

Steward of My Spirit Man _____

_____

Steward of My Temple _____

_____

Steward of My Gifts _____

_____

Today I R.U.L.E. over My Life through:

Revelation	
Understanding	
Love	
Empowerment	

Exercise	
Nutrition	
Journal Notes	
Sealant	

God blessed them, saying, Be fruitful, and multiply... Genesis 1:22

December 5, _____ Day Start _____ End _____

My Prayer Focus _____

_____

Steward of My Spirit Man _____

_____

Steward of My Temple _____

_____

Steward of My Gifts _____

_____

Today I R.U.L.E. over My Life through:

Revelation	
Understanding	
Love	
Empowerment	

Exercise	
Nutrition	
Journal Notes	
Sealant	

For God sent not his Son into the world to condemn the world; but that the world through him might be saved. John 3:17 KJV

December 6, _____ Day Start _____ End _____

My Prayer Focus _____

_____

Steward of My Spirit Man _____

_____

Steward of My Temple _____

_____

Steward of My Gifts _____

_____

Today I R.U.L.E. over My Life through:

Revelation	
Understanding	
Love	
Empowerment	

Exercise	
Nutrition	
Journal Notes	
Sealant	

Behold, I will make you fruitful and multiply you, and I will make you a multitude of people...Genesis 48:4

December 7, ____ Day Start ____ End ___

My Prayer Focus _____

_____

Steward of My Spirit Man _____

_____

Steward of My Temple _____

_____

Steward of My Gifts _____

_____

Today I R.U.L.E. over My Life through:

Revelation	
Understanding	
Love	
Empowerment	

Exercise	
Nutrition	
Journal Notes	
Sealant	

The wisdom that is from above is first pure, then peaceable, gentle... full of mercy and good fruits. James 3:17 KJV

December 8, _____ Day Start _____ End _____

My Prayer Focus _____

_____

Steward of My Spirit Man _____

_____

Steward of My Temple _____

_____

Steward of My Gifts _____

_____

Today I R.U.L.E. over My Life through:

Revelation	
Understanding	
Love	
Empowerment	

Exercise	
Nutrition	
Journal Notes	
Sealant	

But seek ye first the kingdom of God, and his righteousness; and all these things shall be added unto you. Matthew 6:33

December 9, _____ Day Start _____ End ___

My Prayer Focus _____

_____

Steward of My Spirit Man _____

_____

Steward of My Temple _____

_____

Steward of My Gifts _____

_____

Today I R.U.L.E. over My Life through:

Revelation	
Understanding	
Love	
Empowerment	

Exercise		
Nutrition		
Journal Notes		
Sealant		

A merry heart doeth good like a medicine: but a broken spirit drieth the bones. Proverbs 17:22

December 10 ____ Day Start ____ End ___

My Prayer Focus _____
_____

Steward of My Spirit Man _____
_____

Steward of My Temple _____
_____

Steward of My Gifts _____
_____

Today I R.U.L.E. over My Life through:

Revelation	
Understanding	
Love	
Empowerment	

Exercise	
Nutrition	
Journal Notes	
Sealant	

The wise in heart shall be called prudent: and the sweetness of the lips increaseth learning. Proverbs 16:21 KJV

December 11,_____ Day Start _____ End _____

My Prayer Focus _____

_____

Steward of My Spirit Man _____

_____

Steward of My Temple _____

_____

Steward of My Gifts _____

_____

Today I R.U.L.E. over My Life through:

Revelation	
Understanding	
Love	
Empowerment	

Exercise	
Nutrition	
Journal Notes	
Sealant	

December 12,_____ Day Start _____ End _____

My Prayer Focus _____

_____

Steward of My Spirit Man _____

_____

Steward of My Temple _____

_____

Steward of My Gifts _____

_____

Today I R.U.L.E. over My Life through:

Revelation	
Understanding	
Love	
Empowerment	

Exercise	
Nutrition	
Journal Notes	
Sealant	

And after the earthquake a fire; but the LORD was not in the fire: and after the fire a still small voice. 1 King 19:12 KJV

December 13,_____ Day Start _____ End _____

My Prayer Focus _____

_____

Steward of My Spirit Man _____

_____

Steward of My Temple _____

_____

Steward of My Gifts _____

_____

Today I R.U.L.E. over My Life through:

Revelation	
Understanding	
Love	
Empowerment	

Exercise	
Nutrition	
Journal Notes	
Sealant	

While it is [still] called Today, if you would hear His voice and when you hear it, do not harden your hearts. Hebrews 3:15

December 14,_____ Day Start _____ End _____

My Prayer Focus _____

_____

Steward of My Spirit Man _____

_____

Steward of My Temple _____

_____

Steward of My Gifts _____

_____

Today I R.U.L.E. over My Life through:

Revelation	
Understanding	
Love	
Empowerment	

Exercise	
Nutrition	
Journal Notes	
Sealant	

December 15,_____ Day Start _____ End _____

My Prayer Focus _____
_____

Steward of My Spirit Man _____
_____

Steward of My Temple _____
_____

Steward of My Gifts _____
_____

Today I R.U.L.E. over My Life through:

Revelation	
Understanding	
Love	
Empowerment	

Exercise	
Nutrition	
Journal Notes	
Sealant	

December 16,_____ Day Start _____ End ____

My Prayer Focus _____

_____

Steward of My Spirit Man _____

_____

Steward of My Temple _____

_____

Steward of My Gifts _____

_____

Today I R.U.L.E. over My Life through:

Revelation	
Understanding	
Love	
Empowerment	

Exercise	
Nutrition	
Journal Notes	
Sealant	

You will show me the path of life; in Your presence is fullness of joy. Psalm 16:11

December 17,_____ Day Start _____ End _____

My Prayer Focus _____

_____

Steward of My Spirit Man _____

_____

Steward of My Temple _____

_____

Steward of My Gifts _____

_____

Today I R.U.L.E. over My Life through:

Revelation	
Understanding	
Love	
Empowerment	

Exercise	
Nutrition	
Journal Notes	
Sealant	

If My people, who are called by My name, shall humble themselves, pray...2 Chronicles 7:14

December 18,____ Day Start ____ End ___

My Prayer Focus _____

_____

Steward of My Spirit Man _____

_____

Steward of My Temple _____

_____

Steward of My Gifts _____

_____

Today I R.U.L.E. over My Life through:

Revelation	
Understanding	
Love	
Empowerment	

Exercise	
Nutrition	
Journal Notes	
Sealant	

Then will I hear from heaven, forgive their sin, and heal their land. 2 Chronicles 7:14

December 19,_____ Day Start _____ End _____

My Prayer Focus _____

_____

Steward of My Spirit Man _____

_____

Steward of My Temple _____

_____

Steward of My Gifts _____

_____

Today I R.U.L.E. over My Life through:

Revelation	
Understanding	
Love	
Empowerment	

Exercise	
Nutrition	
Journal Notes	
Sealant	

December 20,_____ Day Start _____ End _____

My Prayer Focus _____

_____

Steward of My Spirit Man _____

_____

Steward of My Temple _____

_____

Steward of My Gifts _____

_____

Today I R.U.L.E. over My Life through:

Revelation	
Understanding	
Love	
Empowerment	

Exercise	
Nutrition	
Journal Notes	
Sealant	

December 21,_____ Day Start _____ End _____

My Prayer Focus _____

_____

Steward of My Spirit Man _____

_____

Steward of My Temple _____

_____

Steward of My Gifts _____

_____

Today I R.U.L.E. over My Life through:

Revelation	
Understanding	
Love	
Empowerment	

Exercise	
Nutrition	
Journal Notes	
Sealant	

December 22,_____ Day Start _____ End _____

My Prayer Focus _____

_____

Steward of My Spirit Man _____

_____

Steward of My Temple _____

_____

Steward of My Gifts _____

_____

Today I R.U.L.E. over My Life through:

Revelation	
Understanding	
Love	
Empowerment	

Exercise	
Nutrition	
Journal Notes	
Sealant	

God hath revealed them unto us by his Spirit: ...the Spirit searcheth all things, yea, the deep things of God. 1 Corinthians 2:10 KJV

December 23,_____ Day Start _____ End _____

My Prayer Focus _____

_____

Steward of My Spirit Man _____

_____

Steward of My Temple _____

_____

Steward of My Gifts _____

_____

Today I R.U.L.E. over My Life through:

Revelation	
Understanding	
Love	
Empowerment	

Exercise	
Nutrition	
Journal Notes	
Sealant	

For God hath not given us the spirit of fear; but of power, and of love, and of a sound mind. 2 Timothy 1:7

December 24,_____ Day Start _____ End _____

My Prayer Focus _____

_____

Steward of My Spirit Man _____

_____

Steward of My Temple _____

_____

Steward of My Gifts _____

_____

Today I R.U.L.E. over My Life through:

Revelation	
Understanding	
Love	
Empowerment	

Exercise	
Nutrition	
Journal Notes	
Sealant	

December 25,_____ Day Start _____ End _____

My Prayer Focus _____
_____

Steward of My Spirit Man _____
_____

Steward of My Temple _____
_____

Steward of My Gifts _____
_____

Today I R.U.L.E. over My Life through:

Revelation	
Understanding	
Love	
Empowerment	

Exercise	
Nutrition	
Journal Notes	
Sealant	

Therefore doth my Father love me, because I lay down my life, that I might take it again. John 10:17 KJV

December 26,_____ Day Start _____ End _____

My Prayer Focus _____

_____

Steward of My Spirit Man _____

_____

Steward of My Temple _____

_____

Steward of My Gifts _____

_____

Today I R.U.L.E. over My Life through:

Revelation	
Understanding	
Love	
Empowerment	

Exercise	
Nutrition	
Journal Notes	
Sealant	

December 27,_____ Day Start _____ End _____

My Prayer Focus _____

_____

Steward of My Spirit Man _____

_____

Steward of My Temple _____

_____

Steward of My Gifts _____

_____

Today I R.U.L.E. over My Life through:

Revelation	
Understanding	
Love	
Empowerment	

Exercise	
Nutrition	
Journal Notes	
Sealant	

But thanks be to God, Who in Christ always leads us in triumph [as trophies of Christ's victory]...2 Corinthians 2:14

December 28,_____ Day Start _____ End _____

My Prayer Focus _____

_____

Steward of My Spirit Man _____

_____

Steward of My Temple _____

_____

Steward of My Gifts _____

_____

Today I R.U.L.E. over My Life through:

Revelation	
Understanding	
Love	
Empowerment	

Exercise		
Nutrition		
Journal Notes		
Sealant		

It is He Who gives you power to get wealth, that He... establish His covenant which He swore to your fathers. Deuteronomy 8:18

December 29,_____ Day Start _____ End _____

My Prayer Focus _____

_____

Steward of My Spirit Man _____

_____

Steward of My Temple _____

_____

Steward of My Gifts _____

_____

Today I R.U.L.E. over My Life through:

Revelation	
Understanding	
Love	
Empowerment	

Exercise		
Nutrition		
Journal Notes		
Sealant		

December 30,_____ Day Start _____ End _____

My Prayer Focus _____

_____

Steward of My Spirit Man _____

_____

Steward of My Temple _____

_____

Steward of My Gifts _____

_____

Today I R.U.L.E. over My Life through:

Revelation	
Understanding	
Love	
Empowerment	

Exercise	
Nutrition	
Journal Notes	
Sealant	

December 31,_____ Day Start _____ End _____

My Prayer Focus _____

_____

Steward of My Spirit Man _____

_____

Steward of My Temple _____

_____

Steward of My Gifts _____

_____

Today I R.U.L.E. over My Life through:

Revelation	
Understanding	
Love	
Empowerment	

Exercise	
Nutrition	
Journal Notes	
Sealant	

ABOUT THE AUTHOR

Elizabeth Bailey Copeland

Elizabeth is the founder of God's People Ministry, Inc. She has a passionate desire to enlighten individuals of their awesome responsibility to walk in leadership. She is a magnetic presenter; captivating the audience and stimulating action for positive change.

Elizabeth has been successful in partnering with corporate, Faith-based organizations and individuals to facilitate cultural change, acquire next-level leadership skills and to develop a champion attitude.

Her writings include the following titles: God's People: Setting the Standard in the Workplace; How to Lead People – without losing your mind; The Profile of a Woman of Strength; Joy Seekers, I Can't Wait to Have Patience and Wings for the Workplace.

Elizabeth and Jerome, Sr., her husband of 30 years, reside in Lawrenceville, Georgia. They are the parents of four children. Tameka (Cornelius), Felecia (David), Jessica and Jerome, Jr.

CONTACT US:

God's People Ministry, Inc.
PO Box 1733
Lawrenceville, GA 30046

www.godspeopleministry.org

bethempowers@gmail.com

404-899-9801